Sleazy Stories II

Books by Black Swallowtail Publishing

Aaron S. Elias:

Meditation Without Bullshit: A Guide for Rational Men

Aaron Sleazy:

Minimal Game: The No-Nonsense Guide to Getting Girls

Club Game: The No-Nonsense Guide to Getting Girls in Clubs and Bars

Sleazy Stories: Confessions of an Infamous Modern Seducer of Women (also available in German as *Schmierige Geschichten: Bekennntnisse eines modernen Verführers*)

Sleazy Stories II

A Seducer's Sex-Laden Spring in Berlin

Aaron Sleazy

Black Swallowtail Publishing

Copyright © 2018 by Aaron Sleazy.
http://www.aaronsleazy.com

Proofreading by A.S.Y. and Chris Griffith.

Revision 1.00

ISBN 978-3-942017-06-0

To all you horny men

Contents

Preface

Nine years.

Nine fucking years.

The events chronicled in *Sleazy Stories* took place in London and Berlin from spring 2008 until New Year's Eve 2008. I had many more stories to share, but ending that book with what I had, at that point, considered my prime achievement as a seducer seemed like a good choice. *Sleazy Stories* was released in 2009. In that year, I did little more than having a ball of a time, fucking women, and writing about it. In the course of that year, I recorded many dozens of my encounters with women.

My original plan was to release *Sleazy Stories II* in late 2009 or early 2010. However, the problem was that I kept pulling girls and writing those events down. There was just too much happening. My choice was between recording my encounters with women as they unfolded or preparing the material I had collected for release. As you can easily guess, I chose the former.

As much fun as it was to get laid, I eventually had to move on with my life. Still, taking close to two years off, which consisted mainly of picking up girls, isn't what a lot of people can do. I am happy I squeezed that period of debauchery in because that is certainly not something I could do in retirement. As I was working to get my life back on track afterwards — my situation was somewhat comparable to a former drug addict or a felon trying to reintegrate into society — writing took a backseat, and so did picking up women. Furthermore, I viewed it as more important to work on two other books during that time, and I am very happy that I was able to release both *Minimal Game* and *Club Game*. These two books record my distilled knowledge of picking up women. Still, there was so much more material I wanted to share.

In late 2017, I finally managed to revisit my project folder for a sequel to *Sleazy Stories*. I was absolutely overwhelmed by the material I had gathered. *Sleazy Stories II* picks up more or less right after *Sleazy Stories*, in the early morning hours of January 2, 2009. The last encounter described in this book happened on May 15, 2009, and what a crazy story that was! In 2018, you finally get to read about it and many more of my encounters with women in intimate details. I hope you enjoy reading about my exploits. I certainly had a lot of fun researching female sexuality in practice and I proudly, or maybe not so proudly, present to you the highlights of about four months of seducing women in morally loose Berlin, Germany.

AARON SLEAZY

A Sloppy Start of the Year

It's January 2. I get home from an after-hours party early in the morning, accompanied by a young woman. We have sex, then fall asleep. Now it's around 5 p.m. I probably should get up. I turn around and notice a blonde girl whose name I most certainly have not forgotten — because I had never asked for it. She fell asleep after taking my dick. I was quite tired myself, so instead of shaking her and telling her to leave, I went to sleep caressing her firm breasts. That was then. Now she is slowly waking up. I spoon her. She is reaching around, trying to find my dick. Moments later, my dick is in her hands, and she is whacking it. I pull a condom over it and fuck her sideways.

She doesn't come, but I blow a load. She pulls the condom off, takes my dick into her mouth and cleans it properly with her tongue.

"Good morning!", she says and giggles.

I

"Morning!"

"I'm hungry. Do you have food at home?"

"You've just had a load of protein, haven't you?"

She slaps me playfully and giggles, "That's not what I meant!"

"Not sure. I have stuff to do, though."

"Um ... ."

Her expression visibly darkens, but she gets the hint, gets up and puts on her slutty dress. Ten minutes later she has left my place, embarking on what is most certainly yet another one of her many walks of shame.

Clearly, the year 2009 has been off to a pretty great start. Now I'm sitting at home alone, wondering what I should do with my time, so I take another nap. A few hours later I wake up and reflexively get dressed for going out. This amuses me as part of me really wants to stay in. Well, I am young only once, so I head off to Magnet Club, which hosts one of the better indie rock nights here in Berlin.

I should have checked the listings beforehand, because I end up in front of a closed venue. It's Friday, so it seemed reasonable to assume that they would continue with business as usual. I am not the only one taken by surprise. In front of the club there is a mixed group of boisterous British tourists, judging by their accent.

They seem lost, so I offer some advice, telling them about a few alternative venues they could go to instead. Then some girl with amazing legs walks by.

"Hey, join us!", I shout mid-sentence.

LEGS giggles and says, "Sure, why the hell not?"

We hold strong eye contact.

"Let me just finish this here," I say.

"Sure."

LEGS joins the group I just joined myself and stands right next to me. Most likely she is out on her own. With her high heels, she is about as tall as me. She is also smoking hot. I will talk more about her shortly.

One of the drunk Brits wants to find a cash machine, so he wanders off. As it's often the case with groups, dynamics can be quite chaotic. I want to turn to LEGS again, but some persistent girl with a thick Scottish accent and commendable breasts is having none of that. She is tipsy and horny. SCOTTISH is keeping me occupied and not just because my eyes are drawn towards her partly exposed pushed-up breasts. LEGS has her eyes on me, too, largely ignoring the guy who is trying to work his drunk British magic on her. She is clearly the hotter one of those two girls. I certainly wouldn't have minded getting blown by SCOTTISH and covering her tits with cum, but I have my priorities straight, so I ultimately fend her off.

We take a streetcar to Berlin-Mitte and wander around somewhat aimlessly after learning that Kaffee Burger, the first club in the area we wanted to check out, is also closed. Going out on January 2 does not seem to be such a smart idea. LEGS mentions a bar close-by whose name she does not remember, but it is down the street, then to the right, followed by a left turn. It is a place I only ever walked past. The Brits like the idea of continuing drinking inside some venue, any venue, and quickly take off. That was too much chaos for my taste, so I take LEGS' hand and hold her back.

"Wait!", I say.

"What?", she replies, with a surprised tone.

We make deep eye contact. The sexual tension between us is palpable. I don't say anything for a good ten seconds. Meanwhile, she puts her other hand around my neck and moves her lips closer to mine. I'm not going to kiss her yet, though, so I tease her a bit by leaning in and then turning my head with a smile.

"I don't like that bar you just mentioned all that much, but why don't we head over to Roter Salon instead?"

"Um, right. I think that's a good idea."

"Let's go there then."

The Brits are not out of sight yet and we can still hear them.

"Look at us, we didn't even say goodbye to them!", I say.

"I know," she responds, laughing with a very wide and sexy smile as well as piercing eye contact.

The moment I take her hand, all her attention is on me. Well, that is certainly mutual. I also stop paying any attention to the Brits and let them wander off. I'd say we are off to a great start.

We are on the way to Roter Salon, which is nearby. LEGS interrupts my small talk by spouting out, completely out of context, that she knows me from somewhere. I find this pretty odd, but she insists that she had seen me a couple of times at Magnet Club back in 2005. I am baffled. Not only is that a place I used to frequent, but the timeline works out, too. I moved to Berlin in 2005, but after about one year I moved to London, and in late 2008, I returned to Berlin. She must have had quite a crush on me. In all honesty, back then I certainly would not have dared to approach her. It's surprising what a difference a few notches on your bedpost make. I stop, because I now remember her, too. I also remember that she used to play a prominent role in my masturbation fantasies back then. Oh well, how the times have changed!

We are in the venue now. We head up the stairs and to the bar.

"Wait here!", she says.

She briskly walks over to the bar and immediately gets the attention of the barkeeper, while plenty of women of lesser physical quality look at her with a mixture of envy and hatred. Two minutes later she is back with two bottles of beer in her hand. One is for me.

"That was fast, wasn't it?", she says and giggles.

"Really well done!"

"I know, right? Barkeepers like girls like me."

In case you are not aware of it, it's a fantastic sign when a woman gets you a drink.

It is time to get things in motion, so I take her hand and lead her towards one of the sofas next to the dance floor. I sit down. She sits down right next to me. Our legs touch and I immediately put my arm around her waist and pull her in.

We are talking about some random bullshit. LEGS tells me that she is working as an artist, so we talk about the difficulties of being creative, which is something I can somewhat relate to, having written ham-fisted poetry in my youth. In more recent years, though, I had a stint consisting of being a muse to young and horny female arts students. Thus, I drop that I used to have a side-gig as a live model, which certainly makes her imagine me naked. Our eye contact gets very intense. I don't pay much attention to the words coming out of her mouth anymore. Instead, I put her legs on mine, and then fully pull her into my lap.

It's time to cash in my chips. We make out.

I would love to say that she is so fabulously good at kissing that my cock is getting very impatient, but the complete opposite is turning out to be true. She is so bad at making out that my rock-hard hard-on collapses almost immediately. If you just want to get laid, this is a bad sign, because girls who have been around the block and are open to random sexual encounters are usually good kissers, due to all their sexual experience. They get literally dozens of miles of tongue and dick in a few short years. (I'm not kidding. Do the back-of-the-envelope math!)

LEGS seems to be surprisingly inexperienced. As kissing her isn't that much fun, we instead drink and talk for a while. Well, she is taking care of the drinking part. Within less than half an hour she has downed her 0.5 liter bottle and two thirds of mine. Tipsy and horny is a good combination.

"Come on, let me teach you how to kiss," I tell her.

"Anything you say, Casanova," she replies.

I show her what she should do with her tongue. She is giggling throughout, but she's a quick learner. Still, I wonder how it is possible that a woman who appears to be that sexually confident is such a bad kisser. (She probably hasn't hooked up with a guy like me before.)

7

Making out with her is now a lot more fun. We add some biting and nibbling as well. She moans softly while I gently sink my teeth into her lush lower lip and pull it back.

It doesn't take long until I enter her pussy from behind with my middle finger, which causes her to kiss me noticeably more passionately. Now we're talking! I'm starting to think that I should seal the deal. In order to give her some room to breathe, I pull my finger out of her dripping wet pussy and back off from kissing her for a bit.

"Fun night, isn't it?", I say, giving my superior small talk skills a good workout.

"I'm really enjoying myself!", she responds and adds, "As much as I like you, I really wanted to go out and dance tonight. Do you mind if I change my clothes?"

I must look confused because she opens her handbag to give me a glimpse of a miniskirt that is befitting a whore.

"Let me change into this for you," she says.

I nod.

She disappears to the toilet. Moments later she is back and I pop a boner when I see her. I already mentioned that she is wearing high-heels. Well, she now reveals that she had been wearing hold-up stockings underneath her jeans. Her tight and skimpy skirt exposes quite a bit of her thighs, and her ample breasts seem to want to burst out of her top. She really does look like a whore. I can't say that I have a problem with that. Instead of dancing, she sits down on my lap. We make out, and I spice things up by massaging the back of her head with my fingertips at the same time, telling her that I will give her a thorough massage later. She gets the hint, but objects by saying that she wants to stay in the venue a bit longer.

We talk some more. She drops that even though it may not look like it, she barely goes out as she is too occupied trying to establish herself in the art world. Such a level of delusion, er, blind determination is much more common among men. Instead of locking herself up in her atelier, she should get a guy with a good job who is willing to finance her. Then, she could dabble in the arts, without having to keep begging her parents for money or leeching off the welfare state. The odds of making it in the arts are stacked against her. On the other hand, with her stellar looks, the odds of finding some schmuck with a fat wallet would be extraordinarily high. She only has a few years left to cash in on her looks, though.

Now LEGS wants to dance. To me, it seems as if she was stalling for a bit, but nevermind. She clearly likes attention. She probably likes getting attention more than getting dick, and I am soon going to learn whether there is something to that hunch. We dance for a while and we are by far the hottest couple in the venue. Some creepy guys ogle her while she wraps her arms around me, pressing her nubile body in that slutty outfit against mine, and nibbles on my neck all the way up to my ear-lobe. That's enough for now, so I tell her that I want to sit down again. In response, she grabs my neck, pulls me in, and tongues me down as if there is no tomorrow. The creepy guys around us keep staring. It is definitely time to get her out of the venue, so I tell her that we should leave. "Okay," she says, but adds, with a laugh, that she wants to change her clothes first. She walks off.

This one is in the sack! I sit down, lean back, and fantasize about how hard I am going to fuck her. I think I'll let her slip into her whore outfit before ramming my dick into her tight pussy. In my mind I'm doing her doggy-style, grabbing her hair with one hand and fondling one of her breasts with the other. I am going to make her scream so loud that my neighbors will call the police.

Ten minutes later, she is nowhere to be seen. I mentally slap myself. She is not coming back. What the effing fuck? I can't believe that I have been played so well. It took me a few minutes to get over it, after having waited in vain for about 20 minutes. I am not saying that I could have banged her for sure. It is only ever sure once your dick is in her. The question is whether she was unsure and eventually decided against taking my mighty cock or whether she only wanted to get validation and did not even want to have sex with some stranger. Her behavior on the dance floor certainly suggested the latter. In the case of the former, sticking to her could well have led to a happier outcome. In similar situations, I ended up fucking girls in a bathroom stall, so this is not baseless conjecture or the dudebro in me speaking.

Life goes on, though. In particular, I don't have the intention of rubbing one out thinking of LEGS. Those days are long gone.

There is no reason to call it a night yet. However, it is around 4:30 a.m. and there is hardly any talent left in the venue. One girl stands out somewhat nonetheless, but only in comparison. LEGS was absolutely smoking hot. I'd rate her a 9.5 on the 10-scale. She could make very good money in porn or escorting for a couple of years. On the other hand, the hottest girl left in the venue is only about a 7.5 at best. She is wearing a black top and tight jeans. Her outfit is pretty boring. Yet, I can sense a fairly hot body underneath her clothes. Her face is pretty, but there is not a single part of her body that compares favorably to what LEGS had to offer. I feel as if a plate with a nice juicy sirloin steak that had me salivating has been yanked away from under my nose, only to be replaced with a soggy Big Mac. Well, I'm still hungry, so a nice burger will have to do instead.

Oh well, beggars can't be choosers. Also, it certainly isn't the case that she is unworthy of getting dick, let alone my dick. Or is she? I look at her, then I think of LEGS again and for a moment I'm considering leaving the venue. Should I just head home? The drop in quality compared to LEGS is too steep. I don't think I can do it. If you're preparing yourself for sirloin steak, you're not going to be satisfied with a fucking Big Mac. I head to the coat check, which is on the same floor, and get my coat. As I am about to walk down the stairs to the exit, the DJ puts on some Morrissey.

It wasn't quite Morrissey, but The Smiths with "This Charming Man." I really like the melody of that song, so I head back to the dance floor. I can certainly enjoy that one song before heading home. I lean against the wall, nodding my head to the music. Then that girl I briefly considered approaching moments ago appears right in front of me. With a smile on her face she says that I should take my coat off because I can't dance like that.

"Why do you think I want to dance?", I ask her.

"Don't you want to?", she responds.

She's turning around, shaking her ass in her tight jeans in front of me. I don't really pay attention. Instead I turn around to leave. The song I wanted to listen to has just ended. I don't get far because she grabs my arm and tries to pull me back.

"Hey, wait!", she says with a smile.

I laugh, "Am I not allowed to leave?"

"No, you're not. You can't leave yet!"

Before I can say anything in return, she barrages me with questions, asking what I'm doing in Berlin and this and that. I still don't really feel like making any effort to pull her. This is a peculiar state to be in because it causes me to say some of the most off-putting things I can think of, such as the following.

"What I'm doing in Berlin? Nothing much. I'm working hard on looking good. Oh, and I fuck a lot of girls."

She looks at me with her mouth agape. The mixture of arrogance and condescension is appealing to some girls, but when I'm in that kind of mood, I don't really care whether the girl I'm talking to could feel offended or not. Then again, it is very easy to pick up a girl if you really don't care whether you'll get laid or not.

The DJ must have made a mistake because shortly after The Smiths, whose singer is Morrissey, he's now playing Morrissey's "First of the Gang to Die." This is likewise a great song. I step on the dance floor, leaving that girl behind. I'm dancing and I'm really enjoying myself. That's such a great song! I don't think of that girl anymore.

The song is over. I hum, "You have never been in love until you've seen the stars reflect in the reservoirs." I'm in such a good mood! I am finally ready to head off. I look up and spot that girl again. She comes over, all giggly.

"I watched you dance. That was so cool!"

"Uh-huh."

"Um, you said that all you do trying to look good. Do you really think you're good looking?"

I let out a very loud guffaw and say, "Of course, I do. Why wouldn't I?"

"I wish I was as confident as you."

"You should try it! Being arrogant feels pretty good."

"I don't think you're really all that arrogant."

"Probably I'm even worse than you think."

She laughs.

I really don't care about fucking her, and that is clear from my actions. Yet, with my Morrissey-infused good mood I think that I may as well see how this will end. I take her bottle of beer, take a sip, put it down, and dance with her for a bit. I spin her around — and walk off while she is facing away from me.

She rushes after me, laughs and slaps my chest.

"You're such an asshole!", she says with a huge smile.

"Isn't that what you like in guys?"

I'm just having fun with her. She laps it up and acts like a kitten that wants to play. I can play.

I walk off. She walks towards me again. I grab her neck with one hand, pull her in close and look her deep in the eyes, but only for a few seconds. I gently push her away with both hands while I smile. For some reason, she is now getting really into me. She's coming back immediately but this time she's hugging me, probably so that I can't so easily get rid of her.

"What's your zodiac sign?", she wants to know.

"Just pick one. I don't believe in such nonsense."

We lock eye contact again. So far I spent maybe ten to fifteen minutes on her. It's been an eventful fifteen minutes, though. It's getting late, so it's high time I make a move. I take her hand and drag her off the dance floor and towards the exit.

She blurts out, "We're going for a smoke now!"

This is amusing as this almost makes it sound as if she is moving the interaction forward.

We sit down on the stairs of Volksbühne. Her hands are all over me.

"I can't believe how little time it takes you to pick up a girl," she marvels.

I think that one is on her. I could point out that it apparently does not take much time at all to pick *her* up. That wouldn't go down too well, so I keep my mouth shut. Instead, I slide one hand into her pants and give her ass a nice squeeze.

"It is absurd how confident you are."

"Mm."

"How often do you do this, exactly? I bet you do this every day."

"Who, me? Nah, I never pick up women. I'm shy to the bone and would never dare to hit on a woman."

Meanwhile, one of my fingers slides into her wet pussy, which causes her to moan ever-so-slightly. Yet, she just keeps talking.

"I have to say that I really don't like dominant men."

"Let us revisit that topic in an hour or so."

"What do you mean?"

I don't reply but shove my finger deeper into her pussy, which makes her shriek with lust.

"Where do you live?", I ask.

"I'm visiting until tomorrow evening. I'm staying with some friends."

"How about you stay at my place tonight instead?"

"I don't think I can do that, as much as I'd like to."

"No problem," I say, as I pull my finger out of her pussy.

She looks at me, seemingly expecting me to say something else.

"You have to take the opportunity. If you don't, it's your loss, not mine."

I say this matter-of-factly. She looks deep into my eyes. It seems that she is getting a bit nervous. I look at her lips, then her eyes, then I move closer and kiss her on the lips. This quickly evolves into us very passionately making out.

We have barely gotten started before someone shouts in our direction, "Oh, here you are!" Now a bunch of people stand around us. She is not in the least bit perturbed by that and starts nibbling on my neck. Meanwhile, one of her friends pulls out a pack of pistachios, so I eat a few of those while I chit-chat with them. She is still working on my neck. From her friends I learn that it is past 5 a.m. and that the club is closing. My girl has to get her coat, so we head back inside. On the way out again, I push her against the wall, attempting to kiss her.

She giggles and says, "Nothing will happen tonight."

"Of course not."

We make out again.

Now we are walking towards her group of friends. She pulls me closer and whispers in my ear,

"If you can offer me a nice warm bed with a blanket and a pillow, I'll come with you."

I nod.

Outside, we bump into her friends again. She tells them that she wants to stay a little bit longer. They get the hint. One of them even wishes her "lots of fun." Her friends walk off. I take her to the nearest underground station, Rosa-Luxemburg-Platz. The next train quickly arrives.

Thank you, Morrissey.

Fake-Relationship Woes

In *Sleazy Stories* you met MAUVE who lives a few hundred miles away but occasionally travels to Berlin, hoping to get some dick. About two months ago, I spent a long weekend at her place, banging her about a dozen times and exploring the scenic region she lives in. I have absolutely no intention to keep a relationship going with her, but if she's ever back in Berlin and willing to hop on my cock, I wouldn't object. MAUVE clearly does not understand what is up. There is a relatively steady flow of emails and messages on Facebook. She also occasionally calls me, but I hardly ever pick up the phone. For some reason, she believes we are in a relationship, which is pretty crazy to me. Well, we presumably are in some kind of relationship.

It's Sunday afternoon. I just sent one of my fuck buddies off and thought I'd relax for the rest of the day. My phone rings. It is MAUVE. My initial thought is that she might be in Berlin, and as I have not made plans for the evening yet, she'd certainly be welcome to visit me. I could not have been more wrong, though. Not only is she not in Berlin, she also seems to object to the idea of adult fun without any strings attached.

After some chit-chat, she gets quiet and asks,

"Do you really want to work on this?"

"Work on what?"

"On our relationship?"

"What?"

She recently spent a few weeks in India on vacation and come back about two weeks ago. For roughly the last four weeks, her messages seemed a tad confused if not downright delusional. I try to clear up the situation by saying,

"You know, I don't really plan things far ahead into the future. To me, things are fine as they are right now."

"I noticed you barely respond to my emails."

"I check my emails every few days or so. What's the matter?"

"It's just that I thought you should be more involved."

Now she is getting on my nerves. There is the problem that it is not uncommon for women to dislike not having a boyfriend, and if they don't have a boyfriend, they fantasize that whomever they are currently fucking (or not) is somehow their boyfriend. In my case, I apparently got the supposed-boyfriend status because I fucked her a few times last autumn, and occasionally send brief responses to her emails. Yet, it has been many weeks since I last had my dick in her. I just engage her in conversation every once in a while because I see some convenience in her dropping by and hopping on my dick.

Her tone suddenly changes.

"I checked your Facebook page."

"Okay."

"I saw that some girl had tagged you in a picture, but that tag disappeared a few hours later. It looked as if you two were making out."

"Probably some girl I met."

"I really don't know ... ."

I have enough of this nonsense, so I interrupt her.

"No, I really don't know what you are harping on about. We are not in a relationship, and as far as I am concerned, you're welcome to come over if you're around, but if this doesn't happen, then so be it."

"So, what about that other girl?"

"I think we are completely talking past each other."

Silence.

I tell her that I have stuff to do and hang up. Some women are crazy.

Thirty minutes later she calls again, but I don't pick up. The next time I look at my phone, I notice an insanely long text message, starting with, "Now that I know that you don't like checking your emails ... ." My eyes are getting wider and wider as I scroll down, because there is no way she is mentally stable. I don't think I ever hit the 140 character limit of an SMS message, while she dropped probably well in excess of 140 *words* on me. I quote the key part: "I have thought long and hard about our last telephone conversation. It seemed you were disappointed that I would not come to Berlin before February. Apparently, we have different expectations and I'd like us to talk about it."

This is getting ridiculous. It seems that MAUVE lives in a parallel reality where I am chasing her. I've had my fill of her bullshit for the day, so I delete the novella she sent me.

Fast forward to next weekend. My phone is vibrating on Saturday at around 10:00 a.m. This wakes me up, and the girl sleeping next to me as well.

"Who's calling you at such an ungodly hour?"

"I don't care."

I turn off my phone and turn my attention to my blonde

bombshell of a fuck buddy, putting my morning wood to good use. Then we nap some more. A few hours later we finally get out of bed. My phone rings again.

"Don't worry, take it. I'll need some time in the bathroom anyway," my female fuck toy states.

It's deranged Mauve again. She greets me with, "I don't want to continue our relationship."

What the hell? I am the one not giving a damn about our supposed relationship, and now she wants to frame it as if I desperately want to keep this thing going while she really was never all that interested. Of course.

"Bummer," I dryly say and roll my eyes.

"Listen, Aaron, I really like you, but I am looking for something else. Fidelity is very important to me, and there are too many stories you have not properly explained to me."

I nod but don't say anything.

What would come out of her mouth now, though, was some of the most illogical reasoning I have ever heard from a woman, and that means something.

"As I looked through your Facebook profile, I discovered a few suspicious comments by other girls, which makes me very uncomfortable."

"I am fully aware that I am not what you are looking for, and I never was. I really don't know what you are harping on about."

Now she's silent. After half a minute of this, I tell her that I'm going to hang up.

"Have a nice day," I say.

"No, don't do that!"

"Why?"

"There is something else I have to say."

"Okay, but make it quick."

"When I was in India, I, I ... ."

"Yes?"

"There was that one guy ... ."

"That's fine, really."

"But it's *not fine* because if I am really in love with someone, I am faithful. It's just that I got bored on that beach, and then there was this guy, and then things just kind of happened."

She sounds really upset.

"I don't think I need to hear that."

"No, you have to hear it! Because me having sex with this guy proves, it totally proves, that I can't have been in love with you. This couldn't have happened in that case. If I had been in love with you I wouldn't have had sex with him because I'm faithful."

Listening to this is making my head hurt, but she does not stop.

"We never really were compatible anyway. We are extremely different, always were, and always will be!"

"Okay."

"But I really like you and think we should stay friends."

"If you say so."

"But when I'm back in Berlin in February, I do not want to see you."

"I understand."

She seems to have a need to unload. Now she's again talking about faithfulness, and about the kind of guy she really deserves.

I snap and say, "Listen, what you are looking for does not exist. To be completely blunt, you made a huge fucking mistake when you left your boyfriend. How long were you two together, seven years? How much luck did you have with guys since then? Was there anyone who seemed seriously interested in you? Or even just remotely? If memory serves me right, you said that the guys you meet are struggling with commitment. Maybe *they* are just looking for something else."

A long pause ensues. Her voice gets brittle and she protests like a stupid little girl, telling me, "Of course true love exists! I was together with my ex-boyfriend for seven years."

"And then you left him on a whim because you thought you deserve someone better."

She does not take this well. I hear nothing for a while, then I hear her sob. After a pause, she tells me that she has to get going, and, strangely enough, reiterates that she really likes me, adding, "maybe we can meet for coffee when I am in Berlin next time."

I hang up.

A few minutes later, my fuck buddy comes back, asking whom I was talking to. I give her a brief summary, and she chimes in,

"It is really nice of you that you talked to her. I think she doesn't understand that a guy like you is not suitable for a relationship, but you sure are a great placeholder until my next boyfriend comes along."

She grabs my crotch, to which my dick responds positively. Then she pulls my sweatpants down and takes my dick in her mouth.[1]

---

[1] MAUVE did not do so well. When I met her, she confidently told me, quoting from the movie *Good Will Hunting*, "I put my money back on the table, see what kind of cards I get." That referred both to her career and her relationship. She had left her long-term boyfriend and handed in her resignation letter at work, without having lined up a new job. That move did not seem very

convincing back then either. From what I gather, she ended up as a cat lady in her late 30s. Her career went nowhere, but she sure tries making her humdrum job sound glamorous on LinkedIn. Thus, instead of having it all, a great career and the ideal husband, she ended up with nothing in the end. She got what she deserved.

My First Stripper

The other day NERO hit me up. He is one of my local acquaintances in Berlin. NERO gets laid quite a bit, which is in no small part due to him being in shape, making a lot of money, and living in a swanky penthouse. He worked hard in his twenties, and now, in his late 30s, he's enjoying the fruits of his labor. We chatted for a bit and agreed on going out sometime soon.

It's Thursday afternoon and I am heading home from banging one of my friends with benefits. My phone rings. It is NERO.

"Hey mate, I'm working from home tomorrow. How about we head to Sage tonight?"

Sage is a rock club that draws a rather varied crowd. It's a pretty big place, so it is difficult to run out of attractive women to hit on. I agree and tell him I'll meet him there tonight. Minutes later BYTE calls me on the phone. He's officially working on his startup but seems to spend more time on banging women. We went out last week, and we both pulled. He's doing very well on his own, but thanks to one or two pointers I gave him, he managed to pull his chick a lot sooner than he otherwise would have. BYTE asks if I'm going out, so I invited him to come along.

This being Berlin, I show up late. At 1:45 a.m. I finally get in, after half an hour or so in the queue. It has been a while since I last went to Sage. While I remembered the place having a quite favorable male-to-female ratio, that does not yet seem to be the case tonight. I notice quite a few seemingly aggressive guys, the kind who are happy to try to provoke you into a fight. They have three dance floors, and I don't really like any of those. I also notice that I stick out like a sore thumb because I certainly don't look as if I listen to hard rock. Well, that's because I don't.

I'm still looking for the coat check as I bump into BYTE. He is already working on a girl who seems ready to leave the venue with him. I do not want to slow down his progress and delay getting his dick wet with her, so we just briefly speak to each other. As I turn around to leave, I gently push his girl towards him. She giggles and ends up wrapping her arms around his neck and licking his ear. We high-five each other. Then I'm on my own again.

A few minutes later I finally bump into NERO. We chat

for a bit, but then there is this cute Asian girl walking past us. I stop mid-sentence and stare at her. NERO laughs.

"We'll continue later. Now I have something to take care off," I say as I turn away.

"No worries, man!"

Compared to hanging out with guys who don't get laid, NERO knows what's up and just lets me do my thing.

I walk up to the Asian girl and say, "You're really hot!"

"I think you are very attractive, too."

"Now that we settled this ... ," I say and lean in to kiss her.

She giggles, puts both hands on my chest and gently pushes me away, but not very convincingly.

"You're really funny, but you'll have to look for some other girl tonight."

"I don't think I have to look any further."

"No, seriously. I know you're a player. I don't judge you, but I don't think I should get involved with a guy like you."

"Oh, I think you totally should," I say and pull her in. She giggles again.

"Okay, time out! I'm here with colleagues from work. We are on a business trip. I'm only in this place because

I kind of have to. You know, it's peer pressure. Besides, I have a husband and kids back home," she says while laughing.

"Oh! How old are you, anyway?"

"I turned forty last month."

I look at her, with my mouth agape.

"No fucking way you're forty years old!"

She feels flattered by that, so she shows me her passport. It is true.

"Okay, player! It was really fun meeting you, but you should not waste your time with me."

We hug and I walk off. At the ripe old age of forty, this Hong Kongese woman manages to look younger than many Western women in their mid-twenties.

I walk up to the next girl. She tells me that I'm hot and that if she didn't have a boyfriend, she would "totally let me pick her up."

While those two interactions were not unpleasant, they did not get me any closer to getting my rocks off. Maybe it's time to check out the dance floors. I walk towards the stairs to the more intimate lower dance floor. On the way there, some guy points at my Rolling Stones T-shirt and says, "Dude, great timing! They are playing one of their songs downstairs right now." That wasn't quite right, though, because the song the DJ is playing is "I was made for loving you" by KISS.

It's not going too well for me at first. There is not a single girl who is showing particular interest. Not for long, though, because there is now a group of two girls in front of me. The girl I find more attractive does not seem particularly interested. Her friend, on the other hand, thought that I'm a great match for her. "I'll leave you two alone for a while," she says, before disappearing towards the bar. The girl I am now stuck with seems to be a bit difficult. Judging by how she is looking at me, she is clearly into me. Yet, I just can't get her to warm up, which eventually I put down to her being rather young and inexperienced. After a few slightly awkward minutes she tells me that she has to go to the toilet.

For lack of a better option, I lean against the wall and bop my head to the music. Minutes later two new girls show up. One of them is quite tall and dressed completely in white, which is a rather peculiar choice for a grimy rock club, but arguably an excellent choice to get noticed. The other is really short and wears very tight trousers and a similarly tight polka-dotted top from which her most likely fake tits are trying hard to get out of. DOTS looks like a real-life sex doll with her height of about 5 feet, hair extensions, and heavy makeup. I move closer to her. She moves away a bit. I try taking her hand. She pulls it back. Meanwhile, she gives me this piercing look. Okay, I'll keep going then.

My next move is a hip bump. Yet, DOTS is not having any of this and steps sideways — and smiles mischievously at me. I can play games too, so I turn my attention to her friend. WHITE turns out to be a very cool girl and is overly eager to talk to me. She is not afraid to tease me, either.

"How come you do the limp wrist? You aren't gay, are you?", she asks.

"Yeah, I'm pretty sure I'm not."

"It doesn't really matter either way. I've fucked a few gay guys. You can say what you want, to me you look gay."

"I thought it didn't matter."

She giggles. We share some very intense eye contact.

"No, really. Are you aware of how you dance?", she asks.

She parodies my movements on the dance floor, doing some very exaggerated gyrations with her hips. Eventually, she throws her arms around me and starts laughing. We both laugh for a while.

DOTS apparently does not like getting ignored. Shortly after WHITE has given me some room to breathe, she moves very close to me. Now she is grinding sideways into me, first very hesitantly and gently, but after a few attempts, and after I bend my knees a bit so that her firm ass can reach my crotch, with quite some zest. I'm getting hard, and not just because I'm getting a closer look at her big tits, which are popping out of her top.

A dude shows up. Let's call him FatRocker.

"You got a great T-shirt," he says to me.

"Thanks! Yours isn't that bad either. But why the fuck do you walk around with a print of a dildo?"

Everybody laughs, including FatRocker. No, he did not walk around with a print of a dildo. However, the symbol on his T-shirt is vaguely phallic.

"I got this at New Zealand's most famous tattoo studio," he lectures me.

"How many tattoo studios are in that country?"

We laugh again. In all seriousness, I don't think it would have been much of a brag if he had walked around with a T-shirt bought at Europe's or the United States' self-declared most famous tattoo studio.

"I don't know. But I kinda traveled to the end of the world to get it."

"I would have done the same!"

"Really?"

"Totally."

Of course I'm not serious. However, that is enough bullshitting to break the ice. Now we are best friends. Well, not really. FatRocker turns to White, probably hitting on her. That's great because I can now continue working on Dots. I'm in a pretty good situation because her friend clearly likes me and she now also has a dude to have fun with.

I turn to Dots, take her hand, spin her around, and pull her in. As she seems very compliant, I am curious to see what will happen. Dots has some crazy moves in her repertoire. Suddenly, she jumps up and puts her left leg, fully stretched out, against my shoulder. The other leg is also stretched, so it looks like she is doing the splits, toes on the group, the other leg against my shoulder. I take her by the waist with both hands and slowly lift her up, well over my head. She must weigh only around 90 pounds, which makes this very easy to do.

I think this is crazy enough. I still hold her up by her waist. Now she is spreading her legs so that they form a straight line. I lower her a little bit, causing her crotch to be right in front of my face. Then I put her down. I'm really impressed by how strong and flexible she is, so I ask her,

"Where did you learn all that?"

"Oh, that? My parents put me into ballet class when I was four, did that for ten years or so, and then I moved on to acrobatic dancing."

"I'm really impressed."

"Yeah, I like dancing. I'm also very good with the pole."

"You mean you strip?"

Now a random girl intervenes, all giggly and telling us that we were amazing on the dance floor.

"Are you guys in *Dirty Dancing*?", she wants to know.

She is not talking about the movie but about a dance performance that is about to open in Berlin.

"Yeah, we are," I bullshit.

"That is so cool! I can't wait to see you on stage," she says and shrieks, and walks away.

"You're so full of shit," DOTS says, while playfully hitting me on the chest.

I lead DOTS over to the wall. She stands up on her toes, I bend down a little bit. We intensely look into each other's eyes. The sexual tension between us is palpable, so I lean in to kiss her. She turns her head away, but only to quickly turn it back to me and look deep into my eyes.

I turn her head away with the fingertips of my left hand, moving her hair up and thus exposing her neck. I suddenly grab her hair and gently pull on it. I first kiss her neck lightly, then I suck on it like I would suck her clitoris. She lets out a moan while putting her hands underneath my T-shirt and gently scratching my back. She turns her head around, trying to kiss me, but I move my head backwards. She tries again and I pull back once more. Then I grab the hair on the back of her head and kiss her deeply for a brief moment.

She wants more, but I pull back again. It is driving her mad. She is grabbing my head, trying to force me to make out with her. I push her back while staring into her eyes. She moans again.

"You are really aggressive, do you know that?", I say.

"I know. But it's only because you make me."

"You like to bite and scratch, right?"

Instead of answering verbally, she boldly jumps up, wrapping her legs around my waist. With one hand she holds on to my head while biting my neck hard, with the other, she is under my T-shirt, scratching my back with fervor.

"Ouch!", I shout.

"You like that, don't you?", she says with a mischievous smile.

I put her down again. She turns around, grinding her ass into my crotch, which requires me to bend my knees a little bit. As she is doing that, she is looking around.

"I can't see my friend. Can you see her?"

"No, I can't."

"I want to look for her before we get totally carried away here."

We find WHITE and FATROCKER in the small bar next to the dance floor. There is a bar, but there is also an area that is cordoned off. In addition, a table that got flipped over and placed on top of another table is supposed to keep patrons from exploring that part of the club. The hallway past the cordon leads to an emergency exit. I checked out the venue earlier and remember this spot. It is dark and secluded. Some indirect lighting comes from the bar area around the corner. It struck me as an amazing location for some hanky-panky. Consequently, I take DOTS there.

She seems thankful that we now have some privacy, judging from how eagerly she is making out with me. She's taking my right hand and puts it on her big fake tits. Now that that is done, she grabs my crotch, tugging and rubbing it. Meanwhile, I'm playing with her knockers. They feel a bit too hard for my liking, but visually they are quite a treat. With her other hand she stops me. At first I am puzzled. Yet, she does not want me to stop. Instead, she is rolling her top up, fully exposing her bra. Her big round breasts look as if they are about to burst out of her bra. "This is much better for you, isn't it?", she asks rhetorically.

With her ample assets on display, I free one of her big

breasts from her bra, take the nipple into my mouth and suck on it. She is moaning heavily. Not one to waste any time, she grabs one of my hands and steers it down into her panties. I stop and say, "I bet this is much better for you as well!" Now she grabs my hand with both of her hands, sliding it into her pants. "I'm so wet. You have to finger me!", she urges. She gets my middle finger up her wet pussy and moans. Both her hands are now on my belt, which she unbuckles. I'm fingering her with my middle and index finger. Due to our height difference, this is not particularly comfortable. I'm getting really hard nonetheless.

She gets my cock out in no time. I am so aroused that I'm close to throbbing. I kid you not. She grabs my dick tightly and whacks me really fast.

"Watch it, or you might get a load on your clothes," I warn her.

She strokes me even harder — and then stops, but only to squat down and take my big hard dick slowly all the way down her throat. Awesome! She is blowing me like a pro. Knowing how aroused I am, she holds back, but eventually she starts moving her head faster and faster back and forth. I'm getting close to cumming, but don't want to cum yet, so I grab her head and pull it back.

I lift her up and push her against the wall, pull her pants down, and ram three fingers up her pussy. My ring finger is now joining in on the action. Thankfully we are in a club. Otherwise, her loud moans would easily be heard. She's moaning, scratching my back, and arching hers. I sense that she is getting close to an orgasm, so I stop. We are in a public place, after all.

"Let's not get ahead of ourselves," I say.

She pouts.

We fix our clothes and emerge from that dark secluded corner. WHITE is still hanging out with FATROCKER. DOTS wants to join her friend, but WHITE is too focused on her guy. Thus, this is my opportunity to build a connection with DOTS. How I love doing that! (I hate chit-chatting.) She isn't as uninteresting as you can be forgiven for assuming. We talk about Berlin, what we do for fun, and so on.

"Where do you live?", I ask her.

"In Berlin."

"So do I. We've got a lot in common."

She laughs and hits me on my chest. Then she reveals in which district she lives and even her address. I lift her up, put her down into my lap, and give her a head massage. In between, we make out. She lives rather far away from Sage club, just like me, so going to my or her place would be a bit inconvenient.

"What else do you do, besides stripping?", I ask.

"Oh, I also do belly dancing, but under a different name. Sometimes people book me for private parties, which is quite lucrative."

I bet that belly dancing is not nearly as lucrative as stripping at private parties. (Also, I suspect she's fucking dudes for money.) Too bad I forgot the address of her websites. During our conversation, the fake name she uses for stripping slips out, but when I ask her to repeat it, she stays mum. I don't normally pay too much attention when I talk to random girls. Normally, that's not much of a loss.

Maybe twenty minutes later she remarks that she likes the song the DJ just put on, so I suggest we dance. And dance we did. She seems to have picked up quite a few racy moves from stripping and has no qualms showing them off. After I got the impression that we are drawing too much attention, I'm leading her towards that quiet area again. Now we could continue talking, but Dots feels like having a beer instead, because she is so thirsty. As we are making our way to the bar, White shows up again, eager to share some stories. I let them catch up. I check my phone and notice a message from Nero.

"I'm on the way home with some chick, but let's try meeting up some other time!", he writes.

"Congrats, man! I'm still busy with a girl, but it's going well."

I'm happy for NERO and his triple-digit lay count. I re-joined WHITE and DOTS — and BYTE is with them, too. I see him talking to DOTS. BYTE and I do a bro fist. He says,

"That little hottie just dropped your name, Aaron, so I thought I better back off. I'm not going to mess with the guru."

"Too bad, man. She has already had my dick in her mouth, so you could have gotten a taste of me."

We both laugh. He gives me the low-down on the two or three girls he has been working on. His best lead is a phone number of a girl who said she really had to get up in the morning for an early business meeting. He shows me a few of the text messages she has already sent him. To me, it seems that she can't wait to get his cock.

"Sounds good, BYTE, but how are you going to fit her in with your three or four fuck buddies?"

"Don't ask me. Can I send one of them to you to free up my schedule?"

"I don't know, man. My dad is getting a bit pushy, telling me I should get a job, but who's got time for that?"

We laugh some more.

FATROCKER was nowhere to be seen at that point. He has probably run out of game. While I am catching up with BYTE, DOTS demonstratively walks over to the dance floor, squeezing my ass as she walks past.

"Hold on, man, I have to get back to work," I say to BYTE.

On the dance floor, DOTS tries to play hard to get, but she is not doing too well. She keeps her distance but still makes piercing eye contact with me. After one song I have enough, walk over, grab her by the waist, lift her up, and we make out. I just keep her in the air and walk over to another dance floor. She giggles at first and then sucks on my neck. Her friend is nowhere to be seen, so DOTS does not restrain herself at all. I put her down. First she grabs my crotch, giving my dick a tug through my pants. As soon as I get hard, she turns around, grinding her ass into me. A few minutes later, she takes my hand and leads me to the same secluded area we were in before.

The bar is closed. One of the female bartenders is still around, cleaning up. I nonchalantly walk past her, with DOTS following eagerly. The bartender realizes what we are up to and shouts, "No, don't go there. That's off limits for you guys!"

"Give us ten minutes, okay?", I respond.

"Sorry, that's not how this works."

On the plus side, the bar area is deserted and there is a fairly secluded corner nearby as well. I move DOTS over there. She lets out a sigh and says,

"I really would have liked to continue over there."

"Don't worry, we'll figure something out."

I'm now in the corner, with my back facing the wall. She is in front of me. I turn her around so that she can press her ass against my cock. I put my hands on her flat and firm stomach. We are waiting for the bartender to bugger off, but she just wouldn't.

"Why won't that dumb bitch leave already?", DOTS wonders out loud.

I laugh as that is not exactly the kind of language I expect out of the mouth of a girl. Then again, standards for strippers are probably different.

The bartender does not pay any attention to us. I feel a petite hand in my underpants. She grabs my dick and strokes it. I get rock hard. Meanwhile, my fingers make it all the way from her stomach to her pussy. I slide one finger in, and then retract. I follow this up by massaging her labia, rubbing and tugging it gently with my index and middle finger. With some of her pussy juice added to it, I am doing a pretty good job.

"How about we head over to the restroom?", I suggest.

"No way," she says and giggles.

We continue. She is stroking my cock faster. I put my middle finger into her pussy, which makes her moan again.

"Come on, let's go!"

"Okay."

She is so horny that she takes my hand and leads me there. Things can't progress fast enough for her. We briskly walk over to the big restroom, which has a number of closed stalls. It also has an attendant waiting inside. DOTS does not like that at all, so we head outside again. We head to the smaller bathroom, which only has two stalls, but no bathroom attendants. Both stalls are occupied. DOTS blurts out, "Let's just wait a little."

I realize that we are in a female restroom. That probably puts her more at ease than the male restroom. We have been waiting for only a short while when one of the doors opens. The girl walking out stops, looks me in the face, then down to my crotch, then to my girl, then at my face again. We walk in. Within seconds, DOTS' top and bra are off. She's kneeling down, unzipping my pants. Gosh, is she eager to get my cock out of my pants!

I think there is no reason to hurry, so I lift her up and push her against the door with a loud bang. I pull her pants and panties down with one quick move, and finger her hard with my index and middle finger.

"Aaron, finger me!", she moans.

"You're so good, Aaron!", she continues.

I keep hammering away.

"Please, Aaron, put them in deeper."

She keeps forming sentences, and my name is in every single one of them. My cock is getting harder and harder.

I turn her around, ready to ram my cock up her pussy. Then I look at her and how short she is.

"How the hell are we going to do that, genius?", I say to myself.

There is no way I can comfortably bang her from behind, me with my 6 feet, 3 inches, she with her 5 feet. I bend my knees further, pressing my dick against her dripping wet pussy and slide it in. After a long, "Aaah …" she continues with,

"Holy fuck is your dick huge! Ouch!"

I'm essentially squatting while I fuck her. After a few thrusts I stop because it is just so uncomfortable. I pull my dick out and tell her to take it in her mouth.

"I do everything you want, Aaron!"

I don't let her do this for long as I've been thinking how to salvage this. Sadly, the toilet bowl doesn't have a seat attached to it. I suggest that she balances on the toilet with her knees. That turns out to be a stupid idea.

"What if you keep one foot on the floor, and put one knee on the toilet bowl?", I suggest.

That turns out to be pretty awkward, so we stop after a while.

"Why don't you sit down on the toilet bowl and I climb onto your lap?", she says.

"That toilet bowl? Not really."

"Can't you just lift me up and fuck me while standing?"

"I think you've been watching too much porn."

We still try that for a bit but it turns out to not be sustainable.

"Okay, kneel down and suck me off!"

"Now I don't want to."

"Oh, really?"

I put three fingers in deep and slowly retract them. Then I put two fingers in, hammer her G-spot like a maniac and make her moan very loudly.

"How's that?", I want to know.

"Aaah, aah ... ," she squeaks, unable to form a coherent sentence.

"Now suck me off, bitch!"

"Gladly!"

She squats down, deep-throating me very eagerly. The tip of my cock keeps hitting the back of her throat. I grab her hair and pull her head back. Now I put my hard cock in between her fake tits and move them up and down. She tries getting a hold of the tip of my cock with her mouth and succeeds after a few tries. This is really hot to look at but doesn't feel as good as deep-throating did, so I take my dick and shove it back in her mouth. She eagerly takes it in all the way, while tickling, stroking, or gently tugging my balls. After a while she stops sucking me off.

"Finger me again, Aaron!", she begs me.

I push her against the wall, put two fingers in, and hammer her G-spot. Within not much more than a minute she orgasms intensely, burying her nails into the skin on my back. DOTS is panting heavily but eventually calms down again. Instead of turning her attention back to me, she pulls her panties up again, then her pants, then her bra and top.

"I have gotten all I needed and will now exit the stall," she proclaims.

I hold her back and put her hand on my dick again.

"I was just kidding," she adds, with a naughty grin.

She tickles my balls, then gently tugs my dick. Both her tiny hands are now on my big dick. She speeds up the movement of her hands.

"Do you want to see me blow a load?"

"Yes, of course, Aaron!"

"Then make me cum!"

She squats down in front of me. No holds barred, she gets me close to cumming within thirty seconds or so. Quickly she is moving her hands back and forth while sucking the tip of my dick. I think it's ridiculous how good her technique is. My dick starts pulsating. Of course she knows what that means, so she pulls my dick out of her mouth, but keeps stroking it with one hand. With the other she is grabbing my ass. She is flicking her tongue really quickly, hitting the glans of my cock over and over and over while stroking me. I'm hitting the point of no return, which she immediately realizes and pulls my cock sideways. She really must have done that a lot of times. The precum ends up on her top, but she is fast (and experienced?) enough to move her upper body out of the way, allowing her to prevent that my sizable load further soils her clothes.

She moans while I cum and then says, "I hope you had fun, Aaron."

I'm panting. She moves on to cleaning my cock with her tongue and then puts it back into my boxers. Then she pulls my boxers up. Once that is done, she pulls my pants up and zips them. I laugh as I buckle my belt.

We are heading out. She wants to go first and quickly hurries outside. I exit the stall and wash my hands. One girl witnessed this and stares at me. I leave the restroom. DOTS is outside, waiting for me. It's around

5 a.m. I really want to get going, but she wants to dance some more. She is exhausted too, so she just wraps her arms around me and presses her body against mine.

"Oh, I completely forgot about WHITE!", she suddenly says and adds, "I really need to find her."

We look for her friend. The club is rather empty by now, so if she is still in the venue, we will quickly find her. She turned out to sit at the last open bar. WHITE rushes to DOTS.

"Where the hell have you been? I've been looking for you all over!", she exclaims.

"But I was right here!", DOTS lies.

WHITE seems really upset. She takes my girl by the hand and drags her off. I don't know where to, but as I'm holding her other hand, I'm following. She just wants to leave. Moments later I find myself in front of the cloakroom. I pull out my phone and let DOTS key in her number. Funnily enough, WHITE is now trying to cockblock me. I have already gotten what I wanted, and then some, so I find her behavior amusing. Don't bother, WHITE! Not that she can read my mind. WHITE grabs her friend by the hand and runs off with her. I laugh.

House Party

I have had a pretty rough week. On Wednesday, my kind-of girlfriend stayed over. I told her I don't want to be exclusive, but for some reason she does not mind me fucking other women. Well, it's not my problem. On Thursday, one of my old fuck buddies from London, FRECKLES, visited me as she was traveling through Europe. We did not even manage to leave the apartment. She left on Friday in the early afternoon.[2] Afterwards,

---

[2] Because FRECKLES showed up in *Sleazy Stories*, I'm adding a note on her as well. The last time I looked her up, she was sharing an apartment with two other women her age. They are all in their early to mid-30s, have dead-end jobs, and, with their faded looks, an essentially zero chance of finding a quality husband. On that note, as some kind of Hail Mary, FRECKLES reached out to me shortly after she had turned 30, wanting to "reconnect." That gave me the chills. She was very promiscuous in her prime years and missed the window in which she could have locked down a provider. Now she is paying the price for it. I hope all those years of fucking and sucking were worth ruining your life for, slut!

I headed to my girlfriend's place. She wanted to hang out as she was about to go away for two weeks. I stayed over. Now it is Saturday evening. I just arrived back home and only want to sleep. There is only so much sex you want to have and I have had more than my fill for this week. Alas, the people I share an apartment with have planned a party, so I have to stay up.

You may be forgiven for thinking that if you share a big place with three girls and one guy, you would end up with a party full of women. Then again, my female flatmates aren't all that hot, so expecting a torrent of attractive young women was not my expectation to begin with. So far there are only guys in the apartment. A few of my male friends were happy to accept my invitation. Among them is BYTE, who has been tearing it up this week, yet again. He was very amused when I told him a few juicy highlights of my encounter with DOTS last Thursday.

I also have a bunch of female friends, but I suspect that they only keep in touch in case they get tired of their current boyfriend. One of those girls is DRESS. She's not even that hot. I just keep bumping into her. Whenever I see her out and about, she is either on drugs or drunk, or both. She brought two friends along, one loser guy, and one of her girlfriends. For obvious reasons, I'll call her DOUBLEDS, because she has massive, massive tits. They brought a bottle of wine but wanted to empty it themselves. DRESS asks me for a corkscrew. I get sidetracked, talking to some random girl. When I find them again in my flat mate's room, BYTE is already making out with her. I sit down next to them.

BYTE is a pretty aggressive guy. He just takes whatever he wants. He looks like a bear, which presumably works in his favor. DRESS is a slut, and proud of it, so bringing BYTE into the mix could only lead to great stories to share. DRESS is buzzed already. For some reason she starts talking about dicks, remarking that she has yet to see mine.

"No problem. Pull your dress down and expose your tits. I'll show you my dick in return," I tease her.

"I'm not like all the other sluts you pick up in clubs, you know," she protests.

"Of course. No girl ever is."

"Besides, you are such a manwhore anyway. Getting involved with you would be bad for my reputation."

BYTE and I laugh heartily. Of course, none of that makes any sense.

"How did you meet BYTE anyway?", she asks me.

I tell her how it went down. Basically, we were both out on our own to pick up girls, at a place called Watergate. As a master of that art, you recognize a fellow master. BYTE laughs and takes over the conversation.

"No, Aaron, that's not at all what happened. I recall that as we were taking a piss at Watergate, we glanced at each other's dicks and were so impressed by their size that we simultaneously complemented each other."

That's of course a made up story. BYTE is a bit crude, but his approach is valid because it's quite helpful to get sluts thinking of dicks. He is not done yet, though. In order to further up the ante, he's pulling down her top, exposing her bra. She is wearing some rather elaborate lingerie. Motivated by the sight of it, BYTE slides two fingers into her bra, pulling it down to expose more of her right breast. He is moving really fast, but he is so incredibly good with women that he knows what he can get away with.

"She has very sexy nipples. Maybe you want to have a look?", I suggest.

"You don't know that!", DRESS shrieks, feigning embarrassment.

"Of course I don't, but I'm right, or am I not?"

She smiles and neither agrees nor disagrees. If you're really horny, you could mistake her for a 7. (I've fucked way hotter girls, but she is totally doable.) She believes she is a 9 all the time, so of course she thinks she has sexy nipples. Because more people come into the room, BYTE helps DRESS cover up her largely exposed breast. That was nice of him. BYTE really is on a roll, and

56

says, "How about we have a threesome: Aaron, me, and you?"

DRESS gives us a horny look.

BYTE continues, "Aaron and I would have to share you, but you could play with two big dicks. The only question is whether you could handle it."

I think we are now past the point of just playing around. BYTE has one hand on her back, presumably in her panties, if not on or in her pussy. I have one hand on her thigh, close to her crotch. There is quite some sexual tension in the air. After a moment, BYTE gets up, puts his arm on my shoulder and suggests we get some beers. On the way out, he says,

"Listen, I really don't want to compete against you over some random chick. I can't assess the situation properly because I don't know about your history with her, but I think it would be a pretty close call."

"No worries, mate. I've known her for years. If I wanted to fuck her, I would have done so already."

We laugh.

"Seriously, I was just playing along. You are a guest at my party. Pick any girl you like."

Now the loser male friend of DRESS joins us, talking about some random stuff. Neither of us really listens to him. BYTE's politeness reaches its limits before mine.

He just walks off mid-sentence. I nod from time to time while LOSER talks. I'm trying hard to pretend to be an understanding host.

I do another round through our apartment, but there just isn't any decent talent around. I can't find BYTE for a while but I eventually spot him with DOUBLEDS. He's making out with her! I have to laugh. BYTE sees me and waves me over. DOUBLEDS seems very excited to talk to me and tells me that she just recalled that she has seen me two years ago or so once when I had coffee with DRESS. I really don't think I ever had coffee with her. I may have bumped into her once or twice outside of a club, but I surely don't remember having seen DOUBLEDS before. I know I would have remembered those massive breasts. Then again, maybe she hasn't had her implants back then.

DOUBLEDS seems to be really horny. First she tells us about how much she likes playing with her big tits, then she elaborates on how horny it makes her to take a hard dick between them,

"Because when I titty-fuck a dick, I get to play with my tits and a dick at the same time. I think that's so hot!"

I can't believe what I'm hearing. BYTE sits her down on the bed. She puts one hand on his thigh. I stand right in front of her. I squeeze her thighs. Her other hand is under my T-shirt, gently caressing my lower back. As it seems appropriate, I reach into her top and grab one of those huge breasts. My rather sizable right hand feels small in comparison. BYTE does the same to her other breast. We massage her tits in unison. She moans. I realize that there are other people in the room, but they pretend to not notice us.

"You should know, DOUBLEDS, that I can make girls cum with my fingers in no time."

"That's so interesting. How do you do that?"

I remove my hand from her bra — BYTE does not — and use both hands to illustrate how I do it. She gets really turned on by this. I extend middle and index finger, put it on her cheek, and slowly move them towards her mouth. I rest them on her lower lip and push it down gently and slowly. She opens her mouth. I put both fingers in her mouth. She takes them all the way in, simulating deep-throating a dick. I pull my fingers out of her mouth. Then BYTE takes over, seemingly cashing in on me telling him that he can pick any girl he wants, and I don't care. He still has one hand in her bra and now he's pushing her gently back.

"Come on, lie down next to me," he says to her.

"Are you only doing this to impress Aaron?", she asks him.

He does not answer but instead kisses her. They are making out heavily. Well done, BYTE!

I get a call from another friend of mine who has just

returned from a longer trip to New York City, telling me that he saw my email and that he's in the area. A few minutes later we meet up outside my apartment building. I get us a bottle of wine and we catch up like civilized people, sitting on the staircase. It is a bit too loud and chaotic to talk in our apartment. Half an hour or so later, we head back in. It seems that people have started to leave. For one, I can't see LOSER anywhere. Then I see DOUBLEDS who is sitting all by herself, rummaging through her handbag. She's only doing that to appear busy, though.

"Where's BYTE?"

"He's hanging out with my friend in the other room."

"Oh!"

"Yes," she says, sounding a bit disappointed.

I take her handbag, put it away, and sit down next to her. Quickly, she steers the conversation to talking about her tits again. This is getting a bit ridiculous.

"Okay, when did you get them done?", I ask.

"What do you mean?", she says, while playfully slapping my shoulder.

"You know, I'm 6 foot, 3 inches and I really like my physique. I look like a Greek statue, and I can't get enough of looking at myself in the mirror in the morning, which is why I'm always late."

"You are so full of shit!", she says, apparently not realizing that I had just mocked her.

"Am I?", I say as I slide my middle finger down her ass crack.

"That's a really classy move," she remarks dryly, but does not object in any way.

I grab the hair on the back of her head with my other hand and pull her in. Our lips are millimeters apart. The amount of sexual tension between us is enormous. It's too much for her, so she breaks eye contact and says that she has to go to the toilet. I lead her to the bathroom. It is blocked, so we wait outside. I pull her in, she wraps her arms around me — and grinds her pussy really heavily onto my thigh, while softly moaning into my ear. The door behind us opens. I tell her to go inside. To me it seems that it would be highly inappropriate to spend half an hour with a girl in the bathroom, considering that we have around three dozen people in the apartment and just one bathroom.

Minutes later she walks out of the bathroom. I know I have to lead her somewhere else. My room is not ideal because my flatmates stored a lot of stuff in it to make space in the living room for the party. Thus, I take her hand and lead her into the bedroom of my flatmate PSY. There are a few people in the room, collaboratively emptying a bottle of vodka.

I sit DOUBLEDs down on the bed and continue where

we had just left off. The others quickly realize what is going on, look embarrassed and get out. Some random dude says, with a rather passive-aggressive tone, "Do you want us to turn off the light?" My knee-jerk response is to say that it's not my problem that he doesn't get laid, but I don't say anything because DOUBLEDS is sitting in my lap and covering my face with light kisses. She pushes me back and hops on top of me. Now she is dry-humping me. I put my middle and index finger into her pussy and rhythmically massage her G-spot. She moans, pulls my jeans down, then my boxers. She grabs my hard cock and strokes it. Then she pulls my hand out of her panties, lowers her body and rhythmically moves her pelvis. My dick is between her and my stomach.

"I'm so fucking horny," she says.

The door to the room we are in can't be locked. Also, I consider it rather disrespectful to bang a chick in the bed of one of my female flatmates. The one guy I'm sharing the place with, NUMBERS, would be fine with it. Scratch that. I've done that before, and he was fine with it. Banging her there is out of the question, because the last time I checked, NUMBERS' room was the busiest one in the apartment. There's even some wasted dude sleeping on his couch.

"Let's go to my room," I suggest.

"I don't know. I don't think I should even be doing

this," she says while pulling my boxers up. It seems that I have missed the chance of cashing in on her peak level of horniness.

"I wonder what DRESS is doing. Come, let's go find her!"

We step outside into the hallway. The crowd in the living room is dancing and DOUBLEDS wants to dance as well, or something like that. As she grinds her ass against my cock, I notice BYTE who ushers DRESS into the bathroom. He winks at me with a huge grin on his face. I give him a thumbs up.

Now LOSER reappears. I thought he had left already, but he had only left the place to get cigarettes. He talks to DOUBLEDS as she is grinding into me. Now PSY, the flatmate whose room I was in, approaches me. I chuckle at how bizarre this must look: I have some chick grinding into me, grabbing her firmly by the waist with both hands. She is talking to her friend. Meanwhile, my flatmate wants to talk to me. Anyway, PSY is a rather stiff and bitter woman. I fully expect her to tell me that I'm both a misogynist pig and an inconsiderate human being for fooling around with a chick in her bed — even though I had the decency of not fucking anyone in it.

"So, Aaron, is it true that you, er, have done something with someone in my room?"

"Um, I'll tell you tomorrow, okay?"

"No, no, we're having a party. You can tell me! I only want to know if it is true and if so, who it was. I'm really cool with it."

I laugh and point at the girl who is grinding her ass into me. My flatmate laughs awkwardly and says,

"I guess it was stupid of me to ask."

I nod.

I'm pleasantly surprised that she is cool with it, but maybe I'll get to hear something from her tomorrow. We'll see. Right now, I have a horny chick grinding her ass against my dick. Tomorrow I'll think about tomorrow. Anyway, it is time to turn my attention back to DOUBLEDs. We sit down on the sofa in the living room, chit-chatting.

"I really like you, Aaron," she says.

I nod.

"But I'm also friends with DRESS. I don't want to ruin that friendship."

This could have been a bullshit excuse as there is nothing going on between me and DRESS. Then again, I have no idea what DRESS has told her about me. You could now say that DOUBLEDs shouldn't be so concerned because her friend is, at this very moment, banging my friend. Or isn't he? I get up and look around. Yes, there are still people queueing for the bathroom.

Maybe there is something like slut honor, according to which a fellow slut is not supposed to actively try to get laid with a guy her slut of a friend has called dibs on. That does not seem implausible to me.

My interaction with DOUBLEDS seems to be fizzling out. We dance for a bit, but quickly sit down again. She's still horny. When I put her hand on my crotch to let her feel my hard cock, she vigorously squeezes and tugs it.

"What are you doing? Don't make me jizz in my pants," I say as I take her hand away. She channels a little girl and with a deliberately high-pitched voice says, "Sorry," while looking down. Momentarily, she snaps out of it, girl-punches my arm and says, "But don't tell me you didn't like it!"

DOUBLEDS certainly enjoys seeing how much she can turn me on. Yet, as I am getting a bit tired, I am close to calling it a night. She does not show much enthusiasm for my suggestions of heading into my room for a massage, watching some videos on YouTube or to just "chill."

"Why so corny, Aaron?", she mocks me.

BYTE is still busy in the bathroom with DRESS. He's been at it for about half an hour. I take DOUBLEDS by the hand, say that we should check up on her friend. Then I walk past the bathroom door and try leading her into my room. She is not having any of it.

"Really, I don't want DRESS to think badly of me."

I feel a heavy grip on my shoulder. That better be BYTE! It is him. He still has DRESS with him. DOUBLEDS rushes to DRESS. I hear "Oh my god!" a few times, then they scuttle into the next corner. They laugh and giggle a lot.

I assumed BYTE banged DRESS thoroughly, but he tells me that they got interrupted twice — apparently, the door can't get locked properly — and couldn't get down to it in the bathroom. People walked in on them as he wanted to put his dick in her. So nothing happened in the end, largely because people kept banging on the door or barging in on them, which his chick apparently didn't find so hot.

"Anyway, I got to keep moving," he says. He walks off, heading towards DRESS and DOUBLEDS. He pushes DRESS against the wall and tongues her down hard. She was in mid-sentence. Yup, BYTE is a beast. From the looks of it, he's telling her that she should get her stuff and leave with him. DOUBLEDS certainly interpreted it this way as she is collecting her handbag. I decide to act fast, so I take her hand and lead her into my room. There is no resistance apart from her saying,

"You can't be seriously taking me into your room right now."

My room looks like a mess, similarly to a poorly organized storage room. When my flatmates and I were discussing the party, I faced the choice of either agreeing on letting people hang out in my room or use it for storage. I chose the latter. Anyway, I lift DOUBLEDS up and throw her on my bed, which causes her to shriek giddily. I push her down and get on top of her. We're making out heavily.

"I'm not going to fuck you, Aaron!", she whispers.

"I know."

I grab her crotch and massage it. She moans. One of my hands ends up under her top. I play with one of her huge knockers. Then I use my other hand for that, too. I'm working on one of her breasts with both hands. There is enough left over for one more hand. It's ridiculous how big her tits are. I heave one of her big tits out of her top with both hands and play with it while making out with her. Then I put my right hand on her lower back and quickly slide it into her pants. I'm fingering her. She's moaning. I whip my dick out and she immediately grabs it and whacks it.

"We're moving too fast," she says.

"I know."

Of course, it didn't make much sense to say that.

As much as she loves turning me on and playing with my cock, she does not want to get carried away too much. Whenever my dick gets really hard, she stops, and whenever she gets too horny from what I do with her, she stops me as well. I can deal with that. Thus, I just give her some time to cool down before starting over. We go back and forth quite some time.

"Let me get some lube," I calmly announce. That wasn't a smart move. I should just have pulled my bottle of lube out from under the bed.

"No, not yet."

Now I'm kneeling on top of her. She has one of her big firm fake tits hanging out of her top. Her hand is on my dick. Suddenly she jolts up, saying, "Oh my god, didn't DRESS want to leave?"

I put her hand on my dick again, and she gets right back to stroking it.

"Okay, that's enough. You should know that I'm a bit of a cock tease."

"You're doing a good job giving me blue balls."

"I know, right?"

I get up. She's still sitting on my bed.

"I'd love to blow a load on your knockers."

"If you're that quick to cum, I won't be impressed at all."

"I don't fucking care," I say and start jerking it with one hand while I squeeze one of her tits with the other. She gives me a really horny look, which I try capitalizing on by putting my dick in her mouth.

"Wait!"

Now someone shouts DOUBLEDS' name. It's DRESS.

"Shit. Let's get dressed. What if they come in?", she says and stows her big tits away.

"I really have to leave, but give me your phone, and I'll give you my number," she adds.

DRESS shouts, "Where the fuck are you, DOUBLEDS?"

"I'm coming, I'm coming," DOUBLEDS shouts back.

Someone knocks on my door, then opens it right afterwards. It's DRESS. "I knew it, I knew it!", she triumphantly proclaims while I zip my pants.

"How about you ask whether it's okay to enter?", I reprimand her.

At the same time, DOUBLEDS alleges, "No, it's not what you think." At the same time, she's hastily putting her number into my phone.

"I know. It never is, isn't it?", DRESS responds, laughing at her like a horse.

DRESS now hugs DOUBLEDS and says, "I love what huge sluts we are." She is really tipsy. "Aaron, BYTE, come here!", she shouts. BYTE walks into my room.

DRESS hugs both of us, saying, "And I love what incredible manwhores you two fuckers are. Alright, I'm leaving with BYTE now. Thanks for inviting me, Aaron! I hope you've had fun with my slut of a friend." I pretend I don't notice that her speech is a bit slurred. I hug BYTE. For some reason, LOSER now materializes again as well. He briefly speaks to DOUBLEDs, asking whether they can share a cab for part of the way. Now they are on the way out. I lean in to kiss DOUBLEDs on the way out, but she turns her head away. Yet, she stays back for a moment, grabs my crotch and whispers, "Call me. You got my number."

Now they are gone.

It's 4 a.m. There has been quite some turnover as I hardly recognize any of the people in our apartment. It is almost as if some strangers have walked in from the street, which is probably what has happened. I think, "What the heck! I may as well see what else the night brings." But first I have to get some tap water. On the way to the sink, a woman of roughly my age approaches me. She seems really toned, so we call her that.

"Hi!", TONED says, moving really closely towards me and putting one hand on my abs.

"Oh, hi!"

"Um, I think I know you."

"Oh, you do? How come?"

"We danced together a few weeks ago at Kaffee Burger, early in the morning."

"Really? I don't remember any of this."

She laughs, "I'm not surprised. You were so trashed that you danced with all the women in the place, four or five, and then you were suddenly gone. They probably kicked you out."

"You sure about that?"

I did not get kicked out. Instead, I left with some chick. I really can't remember TONED. I can barely remember the girl I hooked up with that night. Also, I don't drink and the few times I do, I drink very little. I am never drunk, however.

"How about I squeeze your ass to help me jog my memory?", I ask.

She giggles.

"I can't believe you said that. But, anyway, you've already done that last time so go ahead, but don't be too obvious about it."

I was just kidding, but, hey, who am I to refute a girl's request? I turn her around so that my back is to the crowd and she's essentially disappearing as I'm much bigger than her. Her ass is really firm.

"My ass feels nice, doesn't it?"

I ignore that. TONED wraps her arms around me.

"Can I get a slow dance?", she asks.

"Of course. It's befitting the music, too."

"Yeah, The Ramones are ideal for this."

We laugh. I lean in to kiss her.

"Oh, I remember *that kind of dance* from you."

She didn't want to make out with me.

"Have we made out before?", I ask her.

"You really don't remember?"

"No, I don't."

"Then I won't tell you."

"Come here, give me a kiss, for old time's sake!"

She laughs but gently pushes me away.

"You're really cute, and I'd like to make out with you, but I made out with someone else earlier tonight already. It would feel dirty to make out with you now."

I wanted to explore that line of reasoning further, but now a guy I remember coming over to fuck my stiff female flatmate a few times barges in. He looks totally wasted. "I'm going to make out with her now," he announces confidently, heavily slurring his words.

"Eww ...," TONED utters and pushes him away, but not so gently.

I laugh.

Now she slaps me playfully on the chest, "Why the hell didn't you do anything?"

"I thought you could handle it. Besides, how would I know that that wasn't the guy you had made out with before?"

She moves very closely to me. Our lips are mere millimeters apart.

"I have much better taste in men," she says, trying to sound seductive.

I lean in to kiss her; she moves back again.

"No, you have to wait! What's your name anyway?", she asks.

"I think you have to wait now."

"Wait for what? Why?"

I noticed two people enter my room, a guy and a girl. I rush down the hallway to my room, expecting the worst. I open the door to a guy with his dick in his hand and a girl looking to the floor, hiding her face.

"Guys, that's my room. Please get out," I say calmly and add, "I'll give you a moment to get dressed."

I do not know the girl, but I recognize the guy. It's RedBeard, the lover of one of my other female flatmates. She is pretty loose, so let's call her Slapper. I close the door and who is standing behind me? It's that very flatmate of mine! SLAPPER asks me whether I have seen REDBEARD. Incidentally, I just have. I tell her to open the door to my room at her own risk. "He might be in there," I say. Then I lean back to enjoy the show.

SLAPPER gets really pissed, barges into the room and unloads on REDBEARD, calling him a "stupid fucking worthless piece of shit", a "mentally retarded son of a whore" and other names. The other girl tries to get out unharmed, but SLAPPER manages to slap her in the face and shouts,

"You fucking cumdumpster! Get the fuck out! If I ever see you again I'll scratch your eyes out!"

REDBEARD keeps SLAPPER at bay, which makes it possible for the other girl to get out of my room. She runs into the hallway, grabs her coat, and storms outside. Man, I should really find a new place to stay. (I have no idea how, but REDBEARD turned it around. An hour later he made out with SLAPPER and dragged her into her room.)

After this intermezzo, I head back to the living room. There I spot another girl, BLONDE. I had caught her earlier furtively looking over to me while DOUBLEDs was grinding into me or massaging my dick through my pants. Of course, back then I was busy, but now that DOUBLED is gone, I may as well see how much BLONDE wants my dick. I walk up to her and ask her how she's doing. "Fine," she replies and adds that she knows me from last month when she visited Psy to cook dinner together with her. I can't remember her at all. I don't cook with my flatmates, and on many evenings I have a girl over.

"Really? Did we say hi back then?"

"I don't remember, but I saw you."

"Okay."

She blushes. That's not something you see often. Or maybe I just bump into way too many hard-boiled sluts. I don't have the impression that she is used to flirting with men. If you ever look for a wife, that's probably a good sign. But she tries anyway.

"You smell really nice," she says and giggles.

"How exactly do I smell?"

She looks at me, says, "You smell sexy," and blushes even more.

"Um ... ," she utters. She has a befuddled look on her face and averts her gaze. Poor thing!

"I don't think I should have said that," she adds.

"No, it's really okay. You smell sexy too. Also, I think you look sexy, really sexy."

"Really? That's so sweet of you to say."

She touches me, albeit somewhat clumsily. The fingertips of her right hand are on my chest, awkwardly tracing it.

"You can touch me," I say calmly as I take her hand and press it against my chest. She giggles. I open my arms. She wraps her arms around my neck. I embrace her.

"I really like your smell," she reiterates.

I kiss her neck gently. She giggles and protests, "This is a mean trick!"

"It's not. You should try it yourself."

Encouraged by those words, she pecks my neck.

I push her against the wall. She gives me a really submissive look that screams, "I'm all yours. Take me!" I go for the kiss. She turns her head and giggles. I do it again. She turns her head once more while she's giggling. I can play that game, so I try a third time, lean in very slowly, and she very slowly turns her head. I kiss her cheek gently and work my way up to her earlobe. She is blushing so strongly that her face is turning quite red indeed. I can't remember the last time I met a girl as innocent as her.

Suddenly some guy shows up next to us, addressing BLONDE with, "I want to leave." He seems angry.

"Is this your brother?", I ask her.

She laughs, "No, this is my best friend."

To me, he is just some loser who does not have the balls to make a move and now that he sees BLONDE getting really horny for me, he thinks he has to intervene.

"We have to go!", he insists.

My girl looks at me.

I turn my head, look him straight in the eyes and sternly say, "How about you fuck right off, buddy?"

He doesn't say anything and keeps looking at me. I stare him down. He looks scared. Moments later he is walking off, with his tail between his legs.

"I can't believe you just did this," BLONDE says, blushing again.

I lean, and we exchange sweet, gentle kisses.

"I don't know why you turn me on so much," I get to hear as we exchange more kisses. This goes on for a while, but eventually, she stops and says,

"I really like you, but I really, really have to leave now. I promised my friend that we would leave together."

We exchange hugs and contact details, and then she is gone, too.

It is close to 6 a.m., and I am running on fumes. There are ten people left in our apartment: I, my four flatmates, REDBEARD, and four more guys and girls. I notice that TONED is still hanging around. She's with another girl. I walk up to her. She says excitedly that I have the coolest belt ever. I think she has a point. It's a thick leather belt with a buckle in the shape of a bull's skull, pointing down to my crotch. Her friend agrees. I move very close to TONED, which makes her friend say that she better give us some privacy.

I gesture TONED to sit down and take a seat next to her. Immediately after putting my arm around her, she cuddles up to me.

"How did it go with that blonde girl?", she asks.

"I don't know yet."

"I see. How many girls do you fuck, anyway?"

"Aren't we getting a bit too chummy here?"

"Come on, tell me!"

"I have no idea, really."

She giggles and then adds, "I can't stay over tonight because there is some other guy waiting for me at home."

"Who said you could sleep over?", I say with a wry smile.

"I could if I wanted to, couldn't I?", she says, pinching my arm.

We exchange numbers.

"How about we meet sometime next week?", she suggests.

I have one girlfriend, three friends with benefits and also said to BYTE that I wanted to go out with him next week, so it takes me a moment to figure out which days would work.

"Tuesday would be fine for me. I don't work, so I'm pretty flexible," I say.

"You don't work?"

"Yeah, I know. My dad has been breathing down my neck lately, though."

She laughs. "My dad isn't too happy that I'm taking three extra semesters to finish up my studies. Now he's given me a deadline. I work on my dissertation every day until 8 p.m. Can you believe it?"

"You'd have to elaborate on when you start."

She laughs again. "I think you're a lot smarter than I was willing to give you credit for at first. Anyway, I can fit in two hours during the day for coffee, max."

"I kind of like evenings better."

"Me t..., er, okay, how about 7 p.m. on Tuesday? 8 p.m. would be better, and 9 p.m. even better. There's a comedy night close to my place. Would you be interested in that?"

"Let's see, but let's do 9 p.m."

I drag her onto my lap. She wraps her arms around

me and says, "So, you're tall, good-looking and kind of smart. That's quite a combination."

"You're tall, toned, and kind of good-looking. That's not too shabby either."

She laughs and lightly slaps my cheek. We hug for a bit, but after a while she gets up.

"Okay, time to get going. I really have to go to sleep."

I lead her outside.

"You know, I really like the idea of just staying over, but it's so late, and my boyfriend is expecting me. I wouldn't want to rush getting to know you."

We hug. Then she grabs my neck with one hand. She stands on her toes, sniffing my neck. I squeeze her firm ass. She gently nibbles on my neck, then bites hard, and finally sucks on it. Meanwhile, her other hand is in my boxers, playing with my dick.

"Okay, I really have to get going. I can't wait to see you next week. Goodnight."

"Goodnight."

I walk inside, brush my teeth, and crash into bed.

Girlfriend No More

You have met CUTIE in *Sleazy Stories*. She managed to kind of get girlfriend status. In hindsight, I think I spent a bit more time with her than I should have, which complicated our relationship. She increasingly pushed for doing couply things, slept over regularly, and also introduced me to her parents. Her mom is just a few years older than me, by the way. I never fully understood why she insisted on me referring to her as a girlfriend since I also made it clear to her that I was not going to be exclusive with her. Strangely enough, she said that this was fine with her. I think she secretly hoped that I would change my ways. Despite my reservations, I have to say that I genuinely enjoyed hanging out with her. I couldn't see myself being in a serious relationship with her, though.

One time, she bumped into me in a club: She is out with some girlfriends. I am out with BYTE, and we both end up pulling. As I'm about to leave with some girl, I notice someone staring at me. Upon taking a closer look, I realize that it's CUTIE. She quickly turns away and scuttles off. I thought that this would be the end of our alleged relationship and assumed that that was enough for her. Far from it. The next day she texts me, asking whether I wanted to hang out. So, she comes over, we bang, and afterwards, while beating around the bush for a bit, she asks me how many other women I am "in contact with." I open my mouth. She hurriedly covers it with one hand and says,

"No, don't bother. I don't want to hear it."

After a pause, she adds, "In the future, I'll just let you know if I'm going out. Okay?"

Nothing was spelled out.

Meeting her parents was a bit strange. CUTIE was 19 and her mother 36. Yes, you can do the math. Her mom sometimes even flirted with me in front of her daughter, for instance by commenting on how wide my shoulders are while massaging my neck. No, I did not engage her mom in her flirtations or encourage her in any way. CUTIE then quickly got up and said "Mom!", in an accusatory tone. She dragged me into her room, apologizing for her mother's behavior, and went down on me right afterwards. It was pretty crazy how good she was at sucking dick.

Where was I? Right, her parents. CUTIE never mentioned her biological father, not even in passing, but her mother had a boyfriend who was the same age as her mother, and he hung out at their place a lot. That dude was a bit of a creep show. Once I was chilling out in their winter garden on my own, while CUTIE spent an hour in the bath to work on her appearance, and he wanted to drum up a conversation about my supposed girlfriend. It must be really odd dating a single mom who has a daughter old enough to have sex with legally.

CUTIE was a bit thick but really pleasant to be with. That sounded wrong. Probably she was so pleasant to be with precisely because she was a bit stupid. She never complained about anything and always went the extra mile satisfying me in bed. Not being distracted by any kind of abstract thought, she clearly focused on what is important in the life of an unintelligent woman. This is at least my explanation for why she could suck dick and use her pussy so phenomenally well. On top, I always fell asleep so easily when talking to her. For me, it was a pretty good deal. I only recall her once giving me shit because I did not want to agree to not fuck other women. She had just squeezed a big load of cum out of my dick with her tight pussy, and I was in bliss. She cuddled up to me and asked me why I wanted to keep fucking other women and whether she wasn't enough.

"No, it's not that," I say.

"What is it then?"

"I just don't want anything serious right now."

She frowns, then she raises her voice ever so slightly, "And what about me? Aren't we serious?"

"Shh!", I say. "I told you what the deal is. If you don't like it, pack your things and leave. You know where the door is."

She looks at me scared.

"I'm sorry, I really didn't mean to. It's just that, that ... I really like you."

That was the one argument we had. The next morning, she woke me up with a BJ, and as soon as I had opened my eyes, she hopped on my dick and rode me fervently.

Five months into our supposed relationship, things got a bit rocky. Her birthday came up, and she wanted me to tag along. Her friends were fairly uneducated 17 to 19 year-olds. Well, what else would you expect? Of course, her friends were about as dumb as her. I told her that I really don't think that was a good idea. She never brought it up again.

Two weeks ago, I stayed over at her place. Because I didn't manage to get up before noon, I ended up having lunch with her family. I essentially got ambushed. Her mother asked me whether I wanted to go on a vacation with her daughter, just me and her. She would foot the bill. "Just fly somewhere nice and enjoy yourself for a week or two!", she pressured me. She was going on vacation with her boyfriend and said that we are welcome to come along. If we wanted to go somewhere else, that would be fine, too. Her money presumably came from her divorce settlement and alimony. From what I could tell, she was only working part-time for giggles. I felt a bit uneasy with that suggestion.

CUTIE later on told me that she had spoken to her mother about me. According to her mom, it was about time we got really serious. I don't want to know what kind of guys CUTIE used to bring home if I managed to pass myself off as a candidate for a serious relationship. In the end, I did not want her mother or rather her ex-husband to pay for a vacation. I most certainly did not want to join them on a family vacation either and made it clear to her that I wouldn't change my mind.

Two days later CUTIE messages me, "My mom insists on me joining them on the vacation. They're looking at last-minute offers."

Hours later, she writes, "We're going to fly to Rhodes. I wish you would join us," followed by, "I'll miss you."

I feel bad for a moment, but not because I'm missing out on Rhodes in late March. You can probably say to girls all you want that you don't want anything serious. They just don't listen and develop feelings anyway.

CUTIE was sunbathing in Greece. A week and a half later, I text her at around noon, asking whether she's now back in Berlin. Unusually, I don't hear from her all day, so I call up BYTE. We agree to go out tonight. At around 8 p.m. my phone vibrates. It's CUTIE! Instead of a cutesy message I see the following on the display:

"I don't want to see you anymore."

That is a bit surprising, I think. Then I think about it some more, which leads me to the conclusion that it really wasn't. If anything, it was surprising she stuck around for so long. As I wasn't particularly emotionally attached to her, that message leaves me quite unfazed. I did not even reply. It was time to meet up with BYTE anyway.

We head to one of those unlicensed techno places. I don't recall the name. It probably doesn't even have one. I catch up with BYTE for a while, but it doesn't take long until we start checking out the talent in the venue. We both decide that a significant number of people must be on drugs. We walk to the dance floor and just stand around. Some hot but trashy looking girl walks past us and brushes her tits against my chest. I put my arm around her waist and pull her in.

"I think we haven't met. What's your name?", I ask.

She says something, but I don't really understand her. However, I understand that she's horny, as evinced by her pressing her body against mine and wrapping her arms around me. She's probably on MDMA. I lean in to kiss her, and we immediately make out heavily.

"I like you," she says.

"Have you taken LSD?"

"Yes, I love it. Do you want some? I have some left."

"Nah, I'm good."

"Yeah, better not take too much of it."

We make out again. I notice a rather large tattoo on her right forearm.

"What does it say?"

"That? That's my boyfriend's name in Greek letters!"

"Your boyfriend's name?"

"Yeah, um ... . Maybe I should get going. I guess it's okay if I kiss you, but I don't want to end up cheating on my boyfriend."

She kisses me on the cheek and then walks off. BYTE comes in, asking what that was about. I tell him and we laugh heartily because to us making out with someone else would constitute cheating already. Heck, I don't think I would accept any girl I'm dating seriously to intensely hug a guy, or even go out to clubs.

I head to the bathroom, take a piss, and head back out. There's the girl with the tattoo of her boyfriend's name again! She eagerly walks towards me.

"I missed you. I missed your energy," she proclaims.

"I missed yours too."

"I know I told you I can't cheat on my boyfriend, but I can do something else."

I feel her hand in my pants. She pulls my dick out and leads me into the corner, which is just two steps away, still with my dick in her hand. She positions herself in the corner. As I'm bigger than her, she is effectively hidden. She has one hand on my dick, massaging it, with the other she grabs my neck, which she sucks on. That's pretty hot already, but it's nothing compared to her whacking me off really fast. She rolls her tight top up to expose her flat stomach. With the other hand, she's jerking me off faster and faster until I blow a load on her midriff.

"I hope you liked that!"

I tongue her down. However, she stops me when I want to shove two fingers in her pussy.

"No, that's too much! I told you I have a boyfriend."

She pulls her top down again and puts my dick back into my pants. I give her a hankie for wiping my cum off her right hand. That was a fine interaction. We chat and make out a bit more, but eventually, she tells me that she has to leave because she has a seminar at university at 10:00 a.m. the next day. We exchange contact details.

We met up again the next day in the evening. I wonder

how I'm ever going to find a wife if all those sluts keep distracting me.

Return to Form

I felt that while I was together with CUTIE, I lost some of my mojo. I still got plenty of action on the side, but because she so overeagerly satisfied me in bed, I wasn't always quite as motivated to pull girls as I used to be. Even worse, I was down to two fuck buddies, of which one was clearly on the way out as she recently told me that she met some guy. She'll probably be back in a few weeks, but for now, the task is to take precautions against a possible dearth of pussy.

Some time ago, NERO messaged me, telling me about a friend of his, BULLY, who is pulling a lot of girls. "You two should hang out. You'll probably get along really well", he wrote. We met up for sushi once, got along fine and agreed to head to a club together sometime soon. That day is today. I get in touch with BULLY. He suggests heading to one of his favorite watering holes in Berlin-Mitte, a *schlager* music party I hadn't even heard of. I can't say I like that genre, so that blind spot can be excused.

BULLY is a really cool guy and pleasant to hang out with. However, he looks quite intimidating, certainly more intimidating than any of my other male friends. I'm on the phone with him. He cuts to the chase right away and says,

"Listen, there will be around 75% women. Are you in or are you in?"

"Okay. What age range and what quality of women are we talking about?"

"You won't be disappointed."

"Sounds good. I have to sort something out first, but I'll call you back to confirm as soon as I can."

I did not miss that he gave me an evasive answer when I inquired about the quality of the women. While I don't mind getting fresh experiences in the nightlife of Berlin, I also wanted to do further research to know what I'm getting into. Online, I came across a few reviews. The rather high proportion of women was indeed commonly mentioned. I also read that the age range is between 16 and 50. That's a rather wide spread, and not necessarily a sign of a club that targets precisely the audience I want to meet, but whatever. My hope was to meet at least a few willing young women.

Ten minutes later I call BULLY.

"Yo, I'm in."

"Great! But let's go there early."

"Sure. 1 a.m.?"

"Haha, no! 10 p.m. at the latest."

"What?"

For those unfamiliar with Berlin nightlife, I better add that it starts to get busy at around 2 a.m. Most clubs I'm familiar with open at midnight, but if you show up that early, you won't have a lot of fun. Showing up at 10 p.m. sounds crazy to me, but it would explain why you find some underage girls there. I think it's legal in Germany to go to a club and stay until midnight if you are below the age of 18. In that case, you are not supposed to drink hard alcohol, though. I have my doubts that in an utterly degenerate city like Berlin such laws are enforced in any way.

I arrive shortly after 10 p.m. To my utter bewilderment, there is an enormous queue outside, easily 200 people deep. The all-female group in front of me notices me. They are all in their late 20s to early 30s and seem pretty buzzed — at 10 p.m.! One of them can't stop staring at me and then turns around to directly face me.

"Hi!", she says.

"Ugh," I think but I say, "Don't bother, I'm gay."

She puts one of her hands on my chest and rubs it. Technically, this constitutes sexual harassment as I certainly do not welcome her advances.

"But can't you just let me try?", she tries to defend her insistence.

Her friends observe her behavior with some concern. That chick seems pretty wasted, so she probably should not be queuing for entry to a club. I banter with her friends for a little bit and ignore her pretty much, even though she keeps rubbing my chest.

"You know what, ladies, I think your friend needs some adult supervision. Would you mind taking her off me?", I plead.

They giggle. After some excited chatter, they announce that they are fed up with waiting to get in. Half an hour is too much for them. They tell me that they desperately need more alcohol in their bloodstream and that they want to look for a bar. Off they go. I start wondering where BULLY is. I can't see him anywhere around. I pull out my phone. He had texted me that he's already inside.

I look up from my phone again. There is a group of five in front of me now, three girls and two guys. One of them wears what appears to be a caricature of traditional Bavarian female clothing, a so-called *dirndl*. I'll call her MILKMAID. I quiz her on her dress. She's not particularly interested in talking to me, but her Italian-looking friend is. ITALIAN tries striking up a conversation with me, with some success. We are still stuck in a queue that doesn't move much, so they eventually walk off as well. I tell MILKMAID to give me a hug, and she very happily complies. I sense some rivalry between her and ITALIAN who eventually pulls her away.

I'm still stuck in the queue. There is minimal progress, but at that rate, I'll have to wait another two hours before I can get into the club. Ten minutes later I pull out my phone and message BULLY, "Sorry, but there is no progress in the queue. I'm off, but I may try again a bit later."

I walk towards nearby Oranienstrasse – not because of the hookers lining the pavement there, but because of the edgy venues in the area. As I saunter along the street and turn a corner, I bump into MILKMAID and her group again. They have pizza slices in their hands. I chat for a bit with the guy seemingly leading the group. We are in the same boat as all of us want to go to a club, so we discuss options. That guy seems like a bit of a tool because when I asked him what he does for a living, he boasted about his MEng and MBA degrees and what a "unique USP" that combination was. USP stands for "unique selling proposition," which is part of MBA speak and describes what supposedly differentiates you from the common herd. I guess a *unique*

unique selling proposition makes you really stand out. (What a tool!) When I ask him whether his MBA was self-funded, and if so, whether it was financially worth it, he bullshits about the "unique learning experience" he enjoyed. Thus, the answer is no.

After befriending the leader of the pack, I'm discussing options for clubs with him. He suggests a place he has read about online, one of those unlicensed and thus illegal techno places. For that place to open its doors, we'd have to wait around an hour and a half, though. "How about we hang out at Tacheles instead?", I suggest, and add, "It's a really unique place." Tacheles is the name of a building that houses an artists' collective that is better known among the locals as a place for easily getting all kinds of drugs. Yet, there are some rather cozy bars too, according to a definition of cozy that includes grime and graffiti all over. Here in Berlin, we call it Berlin-chic and pretend that it's cool. Dirt is the only game in town.

We head over to Tacheles and enter the building via its backyard. On the way, MILKMAID accidentally touches me repeatedly. Ever-so-accidentally I touch her as well. At one point she is about to stumble or pretending to, so she grabs my arm to keep her from falling. She does not let go of my arm for minutes afterwards.

"We should hang out someday," she suggests.

I like the idea in principle, but I like the idea of banging her tonight a lot better. We head up the staircase. My attempt at taking her hand isn't greeted with much enthusiasm. Yet, after we arrive at the cafe on the top floor of Tacheles, she eagerly sits down right next to me and leans against me. The view you have at that place is quite nice. It's even nicer when you're enjoying it together with a cute girl.

MILKMAID keeps touching me accidentally, which is a favor I am all-too-happy to return. Of course, I can't expect her to do anything more racy with her friends or, more likely, acquaintances around. At around 2 a.m., I say to MENG that we should head to that unlicensed techno club. On our way down, however, we get sidetracked. In one of the ateliers, there is a party going on, so we head there. Three of us just walk in, but the guy at the door stops me and demands that I pay one euro each for everyone in my group who just walked in. In Berlin it is customary to pay one so-called "DJ euro" at parties that are supposedly free of charge. With this I have no problem, but I do not like the attitude of the dude.

"You pay now," he accosts me.

"I'm not going to pay for all my friends, dude."

"Not even for ze girl? You will fuck ze girl, so you should pay for ze girl!"[3]

_____

[3] What he wanted to say was, "you want to fuck ze girl." He

"Fuck off! Here's one euro for me."

I walk in. The first thing that happens is that some Brazilian-looking girl just stares at me, and then moves over to dance around me. I could go along, but I do not want to alienate the group I am hanging out with. Also, my intention was to find out about some new places in Berlin. I rejoin my group, focusing again on MILK-MAID. The Brazilian girl walks off, but not without throwing me a disappointed look.

MILKMAID seems to have a problem with physical contact. She even dances with her arms crossed, all the time. I figure I better give her some space. The vibe in that place is a bit too low-key, so we eventually decide to leave. On the way out, the dude at the door shouts at me,

"You will fuck ze girl, you should pay for ze girl!"

I hate it when losers try to mess with my game. That's a typical example of crab mentality: They notice that a girl likes you and because they have a hard time attracting a woman, any woman, let alone an attractive one, they much rather see you not getting laid either.

Tacheles often has some pretty weird characters. On the way down, some random guy barges into me. To

---

made a mistake common among Germans who have a rather poor command of English due to the accidental similarity of the German word for 'want' with the English 'will'.

me, it seems as if he's trying to provoke me into starting a fight. I give him a pat on the back and keep walking, hardly even acknowledging his presence. He shouts some expletives in broken German at me, related to my mother and the size of my penis, but I just keep moving.

We are back at the club — and it is closed. MENG knows of yet another place he has read about online. I forgot the name, unfortunately. It's a proper club, housed in a former cathedral. Their shtick is to be low-key. They are so low-key, in fact, that you can't find the name of the club anywhere in the venue or on their premises. A cool feature of that place is that you have to walk through a 19th-century gate and across a parking lot before you enter the actual venue. In front of the gate I see a girl I used to study with in London. She is as surprised as I am and seems excited to see me. We hug. I learn that she's currently doing a Master's degree at Oxford, and just hangs out in Berlin for the weekend to have some fun.

It's my first time at this club. I was aware that it is a popular venue. In my opinion, the music sucks. What is worse, the most distinguishing feature of this place, namely that the main dance floor is in a former cathedral with an impressively high ceiling, is only a gimmick. Putting a club in there may have sounded interesting on paper, but it turned out to be severely flawed when put into practice. The problem is that the acoustics are really poor. Otherwise, the venue is fairly interesting. Most women are in their mid to late 20s and nicely made up. On the other hand, the guys look all rather beta to me. I hardly register them.

When walking in, two hot chicks with oversized silicone tits comment on my T-shirt. I take one by her hands and tell her that we should dance for a bit, which we do. The other one is fairly stand-offish. The vibe both of them give off is odd. They are probably hookers. I move on. Quickly and quite literally I bump into a woman with even more disproportionally large breasts. Her dress is very revealing. I get a pretty good look at her ample assets and her stiff nipples that shine through the fabric of her clothing. She is very touchy-feely with me, but as soon as she realizes that I am unlikely to spend a few hundred euros on fucking her, she walks off, and straight towards some random fat fuck in an expensive suit sitting at the bar.

Let me go off a tangent: Whores are women, too. I don't often hang out in upscale venues where whores, I mean *real* whores, congregate, looking for customers. Yet, the few times I have had that doubtful pleasure, I observed that they first try to get one of the younger and better-looking guys. Only if those don't seem interested do they try charming the less sexually appealing men. It makes perfect sense because if a whore has the choice between getting paid a few hundred euros and getting fucked by a handsome guy or getting paid the same amount of money but having some unattractive fat slob on top, the former is most certainly the more attractive option. On a related note, I have a few whoremongers among my friends and they tell me that if the whore fancies them, they get better service, which could mean getting the permission to give her a facial, proper deep-throating instead of going through the motions or even anal on the house. But enough with that. I don't pay for whores, so I'll have to stick to sluts instead.

I head to the dance floor, where I spot the group of the girl I went to university with in London. Let's call her LONDON. I wanted to hang out with them, but then one of those big-titted hookers walks over. I check her out and don't mind staring at her even while she talks to one of the male patrons, and then to another one. Those men quickly indicate that they are not interested. Now she walks over to me. She takes my hands, turns around and puts them on her waist. She stands there with her legs straight, leaning back into me, and bending forward so that her tits almost fall out of her top. She's throwing her hair around and shaking her chest. Of course she's only using me as a prop to get more attention in the club, but who am I to deny a young, driven, ambitious woman some assistance in her professional career? I'm happy to help out however

I can.

Meanwhile, the girls in London's group stare at me. Italian and Milkmaid also take note and are visibly uncomfortable with the prospect of seemingly having to compete with a surgically enhanced woman. The hooker turns around, hugs me — yes, I put my hand on my wallet to make sure no bullshit happens — and tells me that she'll be right back. Then she's off, trying her luck finding a customer.

"Do you know that woman?", Italian asks me indignantly.

"Her? No, not really."

"What do you mean, not really?"

"I mean that she just walked up to me. I've never seen her before."

"Oh. Right."

She does not sound convinced. I do not have the impression that she fully grasps what went down on the dance floor and I see little benefit in spelling it out for her. That may have been counter-productive anyway because Italian is now touching me in less appropriate ways. I feel her hand on my lower back under my T-shirt. Yet, I think that if I go for one girl in her group, it shall be Milkmaid instead. There is no benefit in pursuing both simultaneously as this is a rather questionable move, not due to alleged ethical concerns but due to mere practical matters. Let's say I start working on Italian. As a consequence, Milkmaid would be likely to get very annoyed, certainly once I make out with her friend, and could thus very well sabotage my hookup with Italian. You know how the saying goes: If you try catching two rabbits, you'll catch none.

Another reason why I'm not going after Italian is that there is another girl around, whom I find quite appealing: Locks is a fairly stereotypical German girl with blue eyes, long blonde hair and a sizable rack. No, German girls don't all look like that. She also has this infamous stuck-up look on her face, sometimes referred to as "resting bitch face."

"Let me guess, you're totally conceited and stuck up. Am I right?", I say to her.

The tips of our noses almost touch. She playfully hits me on the shoulder repeatedly with a limp wrist, which looks ludicrous.

"I'm not! I'm a really nice girl!"

"Sure you are."

She giggles.

Locks is hesitant to touch me properly, but I feel her fingertips on my thigh and waist. I take her chin with thumb, index and middle finger and lean in ever-so-slightly. I can tell how horny this makes her. The main reason I approached her was that I could sense a lot of pent-up sexual energy. Judging from the looks of it, she's a high-powered and severely underfucked young professional. Her looks are also already on the decline. I'd say she looks 28 or 29. She's still doable, but she really can no longer compete with an 18 or 19-year-old. Still, she looks as if she desperately wants to get laid. I also think that there is a rather sexual person hiding underneath her two-piece business suit.

LOCKS is a little bit tipsy, yet fully engaged in our interaction. She takes charge:

"You're a pretty hot guy, but I can tell that you're way too much in love with yourself. I get the sense that you are utterly egotistical. I wouldn't even be surprised if you were gay and just hit on me for fun."

Well, if a girl accuses you of being gay, then it's on.

"You're right. I'm utterly egotistical, but I can think of a lot of situations where this will come in handy," I say.

I put my index finger on her nose and slowly slide it down to her lips. I pull her lower lip down a little bit. At first she does not know what she should do, but then she smiles and tries biting my index finger. I pull it back.

"Let's calm down for a while," I suggest.

"I think that would be a good idea," she responds, but stares deeply into my eyes.

London walks up to me — or was she walking up to Locks?

Locks squeaks, "Here you are!"

London addresses me with, "I didn't know you knew Locks. What a coincidence!"

"She's an acquaintance from way back," I claim. At the same time, Locks says to her friend that she went to kindergarten with me. We laugh. I think we're on the same wavelength.

"We're just joking, London. I just met her," I say.

"Oh, then you two have fun!"

Then a few more of London's friends join us. In that setting, it is impossible to move the interaction forward. Locks is clearly into me, but in front of her friends I can't do all that much. However, I quickly figure out that I can trace her ass with my fingertips without her friends noticing because we are both leaning against a wall and the club is rather dark. She puts her hand on my lower back a few times. I'm getting impatient.

"Follow me!", I whisper in her ear.

"Give me a few minutes! Just go ahead. I'll join you later. I need to sort something out first."

"Okay."

I walk off, towards one of the sofas in the hallway. Five minutes later I start feeling a bit stupid. I can see that she's still talking to one of the dudes in her group. I walk up to her again, tap her on the shoulder to get her attention and whisper in her ear, "Let's go some... ." I wanted to say, "somewhere else," but she abruptly takes her handbag and walks out of the room. It's clear to me that she wants to be very discreet. I talk to the guy she had been speaking to for a few moments before I excuse myself and walk out of the room.

Outside, I look around, but then someone is poking me in my side. It's her!

"Where do you want to go?", she asks, with a big smile on her face.

"Somewhere quiet."

I lead her to the nearest sofa. She sits down next to me, and the first thing I do is lifting her legs up and putting them on top of mine. As I play with her rather magnificent hair, her hands slowly explore my body, first over but soon under my T-shirt. After a little bit of teasing we finally make out.

"I think we should go somewhere where it's really quiet," she suggests.

I can do that. I thus take her hand and lead her into the nearest bathroom. That would have been too good to be true. As I'm opening the door, she stops me.

"There has to be some other place!", she proclaims, accompanied by quite some giggling.

Her taking my rather bold move of trying to get her to join me in a bathroom stall with humor is a really good sign. We explore the venue and check a few doors we aren't supposed to go through. One reads "Emergency Exit" and leads into a deserted staircase. This seems like a good option. We only have to make sure that we don't lock ourselves out. I verify that the door can be opened from both sides. Okay, time to push on.

As soon as we are in the staircase and all by ourselves, LOCKS tongues me down hard, really hard. Of course I push her back after a few moments because I don't want her to get too much of a sexual release.

"You are everything I'm looking for — except that you are six months late," she whispers.

"What do you mean?"

"I'm going through a difficult period in my life right now and don't think I can allow myself to give in to my sexual desires."

I don't say anything. The fingers of our hands interlock. I push her against the wall, our bodies pressed tightly against each other. I go for the kiss. She gets completely into it.

"You have really nice breasts," I remark.

"I'm glad you like them. Thank you!", and adds, "But you haven't even properly seen them."

I keep my mouth shut. We lock eye contact and make out again. I stop. She gently runs her fingertips over my face and then through my hair. Now her hands are on my chest. Her hands should be on my crotch, if not on my cock, so I take her right hand and try shoving it into my pants. She pulls her hand back.

I pull her in again. We make out.

"Where do you live?", I ask her.

"Why do you want to know that?"

"Where do you live?", I repeat myself.

She giggles. "My place is just a minute or two away, actually."

"Good."

She gives me a horny look. We make out again.

"I don't think we should go to my place. I'll give you my number, and we'll just see. I may be more in the mood tomorrow."

I smirk.

"Okay, I'll give you my number, but wipe that cocksure smile off your face," she says, while hitting me playfully.

We exchange numbers, but of course I am not willing to give up so easily. We make out again. I am very sure that she's really wet. In order to confirm my hypothesis, I slide my right hand into her panties, play with her labia a little bit and finally slide my middle finger in. I push the tip of my middle finger against her G-spot and rub it rhythmically and very quickly, which makes her moan. As I do not want to risk making her cum, I decide that we should cool down again. After exchanging light kisses, we head back into the club. She turns to me and says, "Thank you! This was really nice. Call me tomorrow, and have a good night!"

No, I really don't give up that easily. However, the group with ITALIAN and MILKMAID is nearby, so I better talk to them for a bit, if only to give LOCKS some room to breathe. A few minutes later I turn around to leave that group — and catch LOCKS staring at me. It seems as if she has been observing me. She fucks me with her eyeballs and smiles at me very seductively. I walk up to her.

I know that she wants to be very discreet, so I only put my hand on her waist. She reciprocates. Yet, this attempt gets cut short as one of her friends interferes, telling her that he's about to head off. She turns around to talk to him and presses her ass against my crotch at the same time. Then I feel one of her hands on my abdomen, which she gently caresses. I get really hard. This is happening completely out of sight of her friend.

There are still two more of her friends around, LON-

DON and some other male friend of hers. Both hang out with us for a moment but they eventually disappear to the bar. LOCKS capitalizes on this immediately by grabbing my junk and tonguing me down. She suggests that we sit down. We take a seat on one of the sofas in the hallway, and I quickly pull her into my lap, but not for long. LONDON shows up again. She most likely noticed that there is something going on between me and LOCKS. She sits down next to us. I get the impression that she's a bit tipsy. She starts,

"I'd really like to go to Berghain. I've heard so much about it. Have you been there, Aaron? Do you want to come along?"

"I'm a bit tired. Maybe not tonight."

"Ah, come on! Oh, I never thought I'd ever bump into you in a club. You didn't seem to be the type."

In London, I managed to essentially pull off a secret life as a seducer. Almost all people I met during the day were unaware of how I spent my nights and weekends. Also, the clubs they liked I did not like, so there was essentially a zero chance of any of them bumping into me on a night out. Funny how people's perception differs depending on where they know you from. On that note, recently one of my friends who knows me from partying in Berlin said he can't even imagine me sitting in a lecture hall, taking notes, let alone working on a problem set. Thanks a lot for that level of trust in my intellectual abilities, buddy!

LONDON and her male friend went to the dance floor. In the meantime, LOCKS pulls out a lollipop, licks on it suggestively for a bit, and then offers it to me. That's of course a very good sign. An even better one was her asking where I live. And the best was her response when I told her the two of us shouldn't join her friends to Berghain but do something else instead. "Maybe," she sheepishly replied. With LONDON and her friend out of the way, we have a hard time controlling ourselves. Our hands are everywhere. She straddles me, grabs my head and forcefully makes out with me. I almost feel violated – she's that aggressive!

"If we go to my place, you'll have to help me pick a couple of bikinis for the summer."

Wow, now she offers a pretense for going back to her place! Somehow, LONDON and her friend got the hint that LOCKS and I might not want to join them. They take off, without even saying goodbye. I lead LOCKS to the cloakroom so that she can get her stuff. While waiting she remarks that I am "such a cliche." I smirk in response.

"You are totally the tall, dark stranger. Do you know that?", she rhetorically asks.

I smirk.

"You are also the kind of guy mothers used to warn her

daughters about," she adds, with a wide sexy smile.

I don't say anything, but instead respond with a cock-sure smile. Earlier that night she told me to wipe that cocksure smile off my face. This time she doesn't. Instead, she leans in for a kiss.

LOCKS got her jacket. As she gets dressed, she notices that her scarf is missing, apparently a rather expensive one. What is worse, her phone is ringing. It's LON-DON. This is a make-or-break moment. LOCKS looks at the display of her phone, unsure whether she should answer that call. Then she looks at me, seemingly unsure of what to say. I pull her towards me and make out with her. Her phone stops ringing after a while. I keep making out with her.

"Okay, let's get going," I eventually say.

On the way back to her place she gives me a pretty amusing rationalization for not going to Berghain to-gether with her friends. She says it would be too far away anyway, too loud, and too expensive considering she doesn't want to stay out for much longer. Of course you can't expect her to say that she prefers getting my dick over hanging out with her friends at yet another club.

She stops. I look up and notice that we're standing in front of a large gate.

"Is this where you live?"

She nods. At first, she is reluctant to open the gate, so I kiss her gently.

"Open the gate! It's getting cold."

She does what I tell her to do. Her place blows me away. She lives in a huge luxury apartment: high ceilings, marble in the bathroom, antique furniture, and probably enough space for two families. She gave me a tour the next morning. Now we have more important things to do and head straight to the bedroom. We undress each other like there is no tomorrow. Then she suddenly stops and says, "I really want to get your opinion on some swimsuits." She pulls an Apple laptop out of a leather briefcase, opens it and shows me some designer swimsuits, all costing hundreds of euros.

I'm naked, but she still has her panties on. We're sitting next to each other. She has one hand on my hard cock, stroking it slowly and competently. I have both hands on her breasts, massaging them rhythmically. We briefly talk about swimsuits; I recommend a few to her, and she seems to really take my opinion into account. A warning message pops up on the screen, informing us about battery levels being very low. I close the lid of her laptop and gently push her into the pillows on her bed. Then I pull her panties off, which she accompanies with a soft moan already. At long last, I get to demonstrate to her the advantages of having an utterly egotistical lover.

Successfully Jumping Ship

Last week I bumped into DRESS, the female friend of mine my buddy BYTE bagged recently, as I detailed in the story "House Party." DRESS said that one of her friends is DJing at Cookies, one of the more mainstream clubs in Berlin, and could thus get in for free. She asked me to come along, "because I don't know many people to go out with." (Far from it.) The reason she asked me was not that she had no other friends to go out with, but simply that they all would rather not go to that club. DRESS, however, felt obliged to drop by as her friend was at the turntables. She also knew that I'm relatively open-minded. I did not have anything to lose because if the night really turns out poorly, there will be a few dozen other clubs to chose from.

DRESS arranged to have my name put on the guest list. We had agreed to meet at 1:00 a.m. I show up at 1:20 a.m. and she arrives around ten minutes later, with some dude in tow. She tells me that she met him the previous night. Anyway, Cookies is a pretty pretentious venue. The people seem a bit stuck up. I want to check out the venue, but my phone vibrates. It's BYTE. I walk towards the entrance to get a better reception.

"Hey man, are you up for going out?", he asks.

"You're late. I'm out already."

"Really. Where are you?"

"I'm at Cookies."

He laughs heartily.

"No, you're not. Where are you?"

I tell him to listen to the music and hold up the phone. Rihanna's "Umbrella" is blasting from the speakers. He is laughing even louder.

"Okay, maybe it's not so bad. How's the place, seriously?", he asks.

"My first impression is that the music sucks, the women are at least in their late 20s, there are quite a few couples there and men clearly outnumber women."

"I think I'll have to think about it."

"Yeah, me too. But keep me updated on your plans."

I'm on the brink of leaving. It's 2 a.m. and I think I better systematically prowl this place. On the first dance floor they play cheesy pop music. A woman in her late twenties stares at me as I step on the dance floor. I walk up to her, take her hand and pull her in. We dance for a bit, but right now I'm flying blind. Her dress is not very tight and this isn't the kind of venue where you brazenly feel up girls on the dance floor. There is too much security personnel around to have a really rambunctious party. Thus, I have to lift her up to figure out if she's in proper shape.

I grab her by the waist to which she immediately responds with, "I'm not that light."

No shit! Those older women definitely know how to hide their excess baggage. She has a pretty face, so I try kissing her. She turns away. After some eye contact, I go for the kiss again, which ends up equally unsuccessfully.

"You're coming on way too strong. I think I better go back to my friends," she says.

As she is really not worth pursuing, I let her go.

I turn around and catch a tall blonde staring at me. TALLBLONDE hurriedly looks down to the floor. I walk up to her and take her hand. She is hesitant and says,

"I rather dance alone."

"No, you don't."

I pull her in and grind my knee into her pussy. Moments later her hands are all over my body and she's giggling. She unloads the usual where-are-you-from-what's-your-name-what-do-you-do, which I take as an excuse to sexually escalate this interaction further. She is clearly interested, but seems a bit uptight. Apparently, I'm coming on way too strong for her liking as well, so she tells me that she wants to go to the other dance floor, "But maybe we'll see each other again later." I respond by grabbing her neck and pulling her in. She throws her arms around me. We are making out wildly. I knew that she was just bullshitting. TALLBLONDE is attractive enough, but because I think I can find someone hotter, I excuse myself.

I look for DRESS and her guy and bump into them at one of the bars in the venue. We chat for a bit, but eventually I give in to the temptation of chasing after girls again. First I look for TALLBLONDE and quickly find her. She still likes me but claims that she needs more time.

"I probably need four or five more hours, or drinks, before I am more open to what you want," she insists.

"Let's just see," I say as one of my hands makes its way from her lower back to her ass. She takes my wrist and indicates that I should stop.

"Really, now is not the time yet."

Consequently, I ditch her and walk to the other dance floor. By now the club seems visibly changed. It's a lot darker, the girls are tipsier, and there is a lot more dancing going on. I notice a girl with a pretty great body who is dancing rather wildly. WILD seems to really enjoy the crappy music in this place, flinging her arms around and flicking her hair. I walk up to her, grab her hand and pull her in. She smiles and immediately leans in as if to kiss me. Then she blows at my face, smiles, and gently pushes me away. What a tease! That's a game I can play, too, so I go after her. Her hands are all over my body, and so are mine over hers. As she is very athletic, she makes it look like a seedy dance routine. Quite likely she gets a kick out of teasing guys like that.

After two songs I think I have spent enough time on that, so I take her hand and try leading her off the dance floor. She resists. I turn around and say,

"Sure. It's your choice."

"Yes, it is!", she responds with a smile. I walk off without her.

About fifteen minutes later I come back to her dance floor. Someone pulls on my arm. It's WILD again! "Where have you been?", she asks. I don't answer but instead engage her in another round of her sleazy dance routine, and she's getting pretty into it. This time, she is taking it to another level and blatantly tries to arouse me sexually. At one point I stop and grab her pussy. She looks me straight in the eyes — and grabs my crotch.

We stare into each other's eyes. I rub her pussy. She reciprocates by rubbing my dick through my pants. I take her hand away, grab her by the waist and lift her up.

"I didn't think you were that strong," she gushes.

I smile. I put her down, look her in the eyes, lean in for the kiss, but then turn my head away. She slaps me playfully. I take her hand to lead her off. She follows along but asks,

"What do you want?"

"I just want to talk," I say and head into the hallway down to the bathroom.

"I think I'd much rather sit down by the dance floor," she says after noticing the sign that reads "bathroom." She stops and doesn't want to move. I reluctantly give in. We sit down on a sofa close to the dance floor; she's leaning into me. We chit-chat, but I eventually just rub her pussy mid-sentence. There is no more resistance. We make out.

A little later WILD wants to dance again, which is fine with me. She seems to feel supremely confident with me, so she is teasing me on a whole new level. Her hands are all over me, and they frequently make it all the way down to my crotch. When she feels my erect cock, she rubs it through my pants. I turn her around, but she keeps one hand on my crotch. As I put one of my hands under her dress and into her pants, she jumps up and turns around.

"Don't play with my asshole in the club!", she admonishes me. I didn't even intend to do so.

She shoves one of her hands down my pants. My jeans are very tight, so she has a hard time fishing for my cock.

"Let me help you out!", I say as I unbuckle my belt.

She laughs and says, "You are crazy! Craaaazzyyyy!"

I did not have the intention of pulling my pants down in the club, though. She walks off, telling me that we have to cool down for a bit. She says she has to get a drink. I fasten my belt and dance on my own for a while. Our mating ritual continues shortly afterwards. WILD comes back from the bar with a cold bottle of beer. I take a sip. Then I lift up her dress and press the bottle against her lower back. She shrieks and hits me in the chest with her open hand.

"You're such an asshole!", she proclaims and adds, after a pause, "But I like it!"

She kisses me.

I drag her into the lounge area. I have spent enough time on the dance floor and simply want to conserve some of my energy. To my surprise there is nobody in there. We sit down on one of the sofas. I pull her into my lap. She straddles me. I put my right hand on her waist and my left under her dress. She gets her wet pussy thoroughly rubbed. After a while, I unbuckle my belt and lower my pants. Her dress is positioned so that everything is covered. I pull my cock out. Because the lounge feels like such a private area, I lie down on my back. She is on top, whacking my hard cock under her dress while leaning forward and making out with me. I'd say we have made it past a number of important hurdles at that point.

I don't pay much attention to the surroundings. Neither does she. Then she abruptly stops. Some guy just poked her on the shoulder. She quickly lets go of my dick but remains seated on my lap in order to avoid getting us into a more compromising situation. The guy is PAINTER. She later tells me that he is a famous local artist. I have never heard of him. In any case, I am not very interested in talking to him. He has the starving artist look down pat. WILD claims that PAINTER is her best friend. He asks me whether I'm okay with him talking to her for a bit and is adamant that she should talk with him to catch up. As she says that, I surreptitiously put my cock back into my pants.

I walk around the venue for a bit. When I see WILD again, I stop. She's talking to TALLBLONDE! That can't end well, I think. I walk up to them and play it cool. WILD gives me a rather cold look.

"Can we talk for a bit?", she coldly asks me.

"Sure."

We head towards the staircase and end up in a corner.

"Um, TALLBLONDE is a really good friend of mine. When I told her about you she, er, she told me that you had hit on her before."

I nod.

"But even worse is that she said that before you approached her, you were busy with some other girl."

I nod again.

"I have to ask you: Am I, like, your third choice for a fuck or what?"

"No, that's not really how it is."

"How is it then? Tell me, please!"

"Take it easy. Such things just happen."

"Oh, so you just walk in the club and hit on every remotely attractive girl until you hit the jackpot. Is that how it works?"

She has figured me out, albeit I wouldn't say I am that indiscriminate. Yet, discussing this rationally is not a good choice right now.

"Listen, take it easy. Those things just happen."

"Yeah, girls just jump on your dick without you doing much, right?"

There is no point talking anymore. I take her hand, spin her around, dip her, and then say,

"It's not the case that I prowled the whole club and went through a handful of girls. Besides, it took me a while to notice you, so you're clearly not my second choice, let alone my third one."

WILD looks at me, but doesn't say anything in response. I don't think I managed to convince her. She turns around and walks back to TALLBLONDE. I dance on my own for a bit, before I sit down again on a sofa. I relax for a few minutes. Eventually, WILD sits down as well but leaves a lot of space between us. I get up and sit down right next to her.

"I'm still upset. Do you only want to fuck me? Do you really go from one girl to the next until you find one you can fuck?"

I have no idea whether I can salvage the situation. On the plus side, she is still talking to me, but on the other hand, what is coming out of her mouth isn't overly encouraging. I am not easily discouraged, though.

"Come on now, don't be silly. This is really not how things are," I say to her, calmly.

She looks at me, then she looks away. I lean back. She looks at me again and gives me a faint smile. I feel her hand on my thighs. It seems there is some hope left.

"Sorry, I think I overreacted a little bit," she finally concedes.

"No worries."

We sit next to each other but don't talk much. I put an arm around her and pull her in. She cuddles up to me. With a much less confrontational tone she says,

"Are you really sure you want me? I think you could find a much better fuck than me. I don't think I'm all that attractive anyway."

Girls and their insecurities! I don't say anything in response. Instead, I lean in to kiss her. We end up making out, but much more tenderly than before. She stops.

"Why did you pick me?"

"I like you."

"But ... ."

I don't let her continue and put my index finger on her lips to indicate that she should stop talking. Over the roughly next fifteen to twenty minutes we cuddle and engage in increasingly more passionate make-out sessions. It seems she is ready to forgive me. Eventually, she smiles at me and says,

"OK. I may want to fuck you. But I don't like small dicks. How big is yours?"

I laugh and say, "You've played with it already, haven't you?"

"I only touched it for a little bit, but I didn't yet have a look at it."

"Sure. Let's go somewhere private, and I promise you won't be disappointed."

She shoves her hand down my pants and fondles my cock while making strong eye contact. I don't flinch that easily.

She says, "It's a small one, I can feel it."

I laugh while keeping eye contact. I'm getting harder.

"It seems your cock is of normal size."

I still don't say anything but instead look her straight in her eyes. She keeps her hand on my cock, gently stroking it. I'm getting bigger and bigger. Now I'm rock hard.

"I should stop teasing you. I know that you have a big dick," she finally concedes.

WILD pulls her hand out of my pants. We make out again. She stops and says, "I'd like to dance a bit more. Afterwards we can go to yours or mine, whatever you prefer. I don't care."

At this point it seems like a done deal, but, alas, that is not how things would turn out. PAINTER and TALL-BLONDE come by, insisting that they down a few shots together. I better try befriending PAINTER because my standing in the group isn't what I would call favorable. We head to the bar. I more or less don't drink, so I watch them downing shots. Afterwards, we head to the dance floor, but WILD quickly focuses only on me. We dance very closely. Within a few moments her petite hands are in my pants. She rummages until she gets a good hold of my cock and balls. She whacks my dick, as much as possible given the circumstances. TALL-BLONDE notices this and is green with envy.

I pull off a few dominant moves on the dance floor, which are apparently a bit too much for WILD, given the time. She throws one arm around me and says, "I don't want to say that I dislike what you are doing, but I think you shouldn't be so commanding. Maybe this works with all the other girls you fuck all the time, but I'm different." We make out again. Then her handbag vibrates. She pulls out her phone and quickly walks off. I walk slowly after her, but on the way I bump into PAINTER, so I talk to him for a bit.

Eventually I find WILD in the hallway, wildly gesticulating while talking on the phone. I walk up from behind and wrap one arm around her. She caresses my arm with her free hand, then hangs up the phone.

"One of my friends just called me. She's at Sage. I thought she'll be in Berlin for a week, but she's going to leave tomorrow. I have to meet up with her, like, right now!"

I wonder when I would get laid and whether I should bother sticking around. Also, WILD is getting a little bit tipsy. Right now there is no issue, but I certainly don't want to hang out with a girl who is clearly drunk. Anyway, I embark on what would turn out to be a bit of an odyssey with her. We agree that I wait in the hallway while she collects her friends. Meanwhile, DRESS walks past me.

"How's it going, Aaron?", she asks.

"Good."

"Good? Are you going to get laid tonight or not?"

"Hard to say. I think it's more likely than not."

She smiles and says, "I hope you do. Send me the story afterwards!"

I gave her a printout of a draft of *Sleazy Stories* a few months ago. Since then, she occasionally asks me if I have more for her to read. WILD comes back, throws her arms around me and looks at DRESS.

"We're leaving," WILD says to me.

With a nod of approval DRESS asks, "Is that the girl?"

I roll my eyes and say, "What do you think?"

She laughs and wishes us a fun night as I walk off with WILD, PAINTER, and another girl: BIGEYES, a friend of PAINTER. The club we emerge from is centrally located, so it shouldn't take long until we find a cab. Or so we think. After having waited for a few minutes, there is still no cab in sight, so we walk down Friedrichstrasse, looking for a cab.

"This is boooring," WILD laments.

None of us reacts to her complaint, but upon spotting a policeman, she walks up to him and says,

"Hey, Mr. Policeman! Could you please drive us to Sage Club? Cabs are so fucking expensive."

The policeman ignores her. Then she starts flirting, telling him that she likes to be in a car with a big strong man. She's quite a bit tipsier than I thought. The policeman still ignores her. I quickly drag WILD off because I don't want to get into any trouble. Finally, we are able to hail a cab. A little later we are outside of Sage Club. The guy at the door asks us to pay full cover charge. It's close to 5 a.m. already, however. BIGEYES steps in front of us and launches at him,

"PAINTER and I were here before, and those two here belong to us."

"Oh, it's you! Come on in!"

We walk in. Apparently, BIGEYES knows a lot of people.

Inside, WILD wants to find VIPER. The place is not very busy anymore, so it shouldn't take long. I let her take off. I stay back, chit-chatting with PAINTER and BIGEYES, who turns out to be his girlfriend. A girl walks past me, staring at me. She is dressed like a slut looking to score. WILD is pretty hot, but this girl here is *really* hot. For a moment I consider jumping ship yet again, but that would have been overly foolish. Minutes later another girl walks past. She looks straight into my eyes and slowly rubs her tits against my chest as she walks past. Then she turns her head and gives me a big smile. PAINTER laughs and says that this is really sweet and charming. "You can say that again," I say. The girl laughs as well, stops and waits expectantly. I am on the brink of going after her. I am really tempted. Looking back, I somehow still think I should have. The reason I did not was because that would have turned three people against me, and that could have come back and haunted me.

WILD has still not returned. It has been ten minutes already. I head off looking for her. I knew she was downstairs, so I head to that dance floor. As I look around, someone tugs on my T-shirt. It's her! She introduces me to VIPER and her boyfriend. WILD invites us to drinks. I order tap water. WILD has an arm around me and is in an exuberant mood. I have one hand on her ass and massage it.

"VIPER, I have checked out his cock already. It is — not small."

Both girls laugh hysterically.

I found that hilarious. They keep chatting, while I keep mostly quiet as I am busy kneading WILD's ass. She occasionally turns around to kiss me, presumably to make sure that I don't lose interest. A little later, VIPER and her boyfriend want to leave. We walk to the cloakroom. I'm getting pretty tired.

Out of nowhere, a girl comes running towards WILD, shrieking, "Oh my God, WILD, WILD! Remember me? It's been ten years. We've had so much fun together, haven't we?" WILD turns to me and says, "Please give me a minute. I'll make it quick." How much more crap do I have to endure in order to have sex with her? She gave that girl mostly monosyllabic answers because apparently she now prefers cocks over vaginas. However, when she was back, she said she wanted to have "one last dance." Fine.

Five minutes later we are finally in a cab, just the two of us, on the way to her place. In the cab, WILD pulls a roll of toilet paper out of her handbag and says she does not have any left at home, so she had to help herself to some at the club. As you see, I'm pulling high-quality girls! Seriously, if you think that's crazy, then wait until you hear what happened in her apartment: She opens the door, walks in, and without taking off her shoes, she rushes into her flatmate's room. That girl is sound asleep. WILD hops into her bed and cuddles up to her. I watch this with some consternation. Her flatmate wakes up. She's pretty good-looking, actually.

"WILD, what the fuck are you doing?", she says in a rather sleepy voice.

"I'm cuddling with you, silly!"

"Are you on your own or have you brought someone home with you."

"I'm not alone."

"Then you better keep him company."

"I know. I want coffee. Do you want coffee, too?"

"Give me a moment, I'll join you later."

WILD gets up again, kisses me on the mouth, and heads straight into the kitchen, strutting proudly and confidently. She brews some coffee and tells me cheerfully that she always wakes up her flatmate when she comes home, no matter how late it is, "and that bitch does the same to me!", she adds with a loud laughter. "Besides, it's something like 7 a.m., so it's about time that lazy bitch gets up anyway." We both laugh.

We sit down to drink coffee. Her flatmate indeed joins us.

"Oh, Aaron, do you want some food?", WILD asks me. Before I can answer, she turns to her flatmate, asking her whether she has some weed. I can't quite believe what I'm witnessing. After giving an evasive answer, her flatmate excuses herself, but not without reminding WILD that they should go to the nearby flea market at 10 a.m. Both women excitedly agree that this is an excellent idea. I keep my skepticism about their plan to myself. I don't care much anyway.

At around 7:30 a.m. I am finally in WILD's room. She puts on a nightgown while I undress myself. I notice a big box of condoms next to her bed, the wholesale-sized ones you can't buy in regular stores but instead have to get off eBay. I chuckle because I'm definitely not dealing with a virgin here.

We hop into bed. Considering how confident WILD appeared to be in the club, I expected her to be a rather spectacular lover. That wasn't quite what happened though. I warm her up by playing with her pussy. I put one finger in, then two, then three. Her pussy is really effing loose. I could put in three fingers without warming her up. She does not seem to be fazed by this at all. She sits up and turns around, indicating that I should fuck her from behind. I take a condom from her (half-empty) 144-piece box, tear open the wrapper, whack myself to get a bit harder, and slap it on. Fucking her doggy style in the morning hours after a long night out is more demanding than I'd like. Thus, after a few thrusts I pull my dick out, turn her around and do her missionary style.

After a while she tells me that she can't come from fucking. I like hearing that because I'm getting a bit too tired to have sex anyway. However, because I'm a gentleman, I use my fingers on her, but don't make her cum yet. That takes quite some effort, too. Now it's her turn. I grab her by the hair on the back of her head and introduce her mouth to my cock — and end up getting massively disappointed. Her blow job skills are bad, really bad. The sounds she makes, which she presumably believes would turn me on, are more on the ridiculous side. On the plus side, even though her technique is crap, she's quite eager. She is so eager, in fact, that she eventually teethes my cock. I lose my boner and pull it back. She seems confused by this and asks me what the matter is. I could have pointed out to her how she should suck my dick, instead of her figuring it out herself via trial and error. As I do not want to waste so much time, I tell her to suck my balls, while I jerk myself off. As a reward for her ineptitude, I blow a load on her face, but quickly yank my cock up to target her forehead and hair, and slap her face with my dick afterwards. She wipes her face with tissue paper.

"I want to come, too," she says, not batting an eyelid. Thus, I push her down and finger her hard, using my clean hand. Thankfully she comes very quickly. She screams so loudly that her neighbors can probably hear it. I wonder if there is a competition going on between her and her flatmate, and whether she screams so loudly to one-up her. I lie down on my back, looking up at the ceiling, and consider leaving her flat. WILD is a contender for the worst lay of my life. Yet, I am so tired that I can't help but fall asleep.

Three hours later I wake up again, with a raging boner. Where am I? I look around and remember how shitty a lover she was. Yet, here I am, with a hard cock and a willing woman lying next to me. I check whether WILD is awake by putting my cock in her hand. Judging by her stroking it, she is. I slap on a condom and fuck her sideways. This is good fun at first, but her pussy is so incredibly loose that I don't feel much at all. As a fix, I grab the bottom of my cock and jerk myself quickly whenever my cock is retracted before ramming it into her pussy again. This feels like really awkward masturbation, but with a condom on and minimal stimulation from a pussy. I lose interest, pull the condom off and go back to sleep.

At around noon I wake up again and nudge her. She turns around and immediately grabs my cock. I am not going to fuck her again, though. I put my hand on the back of her head and gently push it down. She starts sucking me off right away. To my great surprise, this time she's actually pretty damn good, largely because she does extensive deep-throating. Apart from that, her technique is just as shitty as before. Yet, my cock likes her throat a lot. I grab her by her hair and

I keep ramming my cock down her throat, and when I pull her head back and my cock out of her mouth, I tell her to stick her tongue out so that I can rub the tip of my cock across her tongue, which she barely moves. She's getting very aroused from how I use her. I'm getting really turned on myself and I end up reaching the point of no return in no time flat, two to three minutes in total. I have both hands on the back of her head and push it down. My cock is completely in her mouth as I blow a load into her throat. She moans and readily swallows. As this encounter ended on a high note, I'm willing to conclude that she's not such a bad lay after all.

We get up. I take a shower, then dress. Meanwhile, she makes breakfast for me, which I find a bit odd. What I find even odder is that she pulls out her phone and goes through an album with pictures of her mother, when she was young. It is full of nude pictures. Her mother was apparently a reasonably successful glamour model in her teens and early twenties. I find it ludicrous that her daughter has taken pictures of those posters and magazines and stored them on her phone. Judging from those pictures, her mother is a notch or two above her daughter, by the way. I couldn't help comparing them.

At 1 p.m. the doorbell rings. It's a male friend of WILD. He seems pretty cool. They chat, and he reveals that he ended up fucking a mutual friend yesterday. WILD accuses him of being a huge slut. He laughs and turns to me, "What's your story, pal? Where did she pick you up?" WILD interjects, stating that it was me who had done the pick-up and then complains, "But he hit on TALLBLONDE before he chose me." He laughs.

As I have some time to kill, I hang out with them a bit more, but after half an hour her friend heads off again. We then head to the flea market together with her flatmate, hours later than initially planned. There, WILD transformed from being a sexually confident slut to a needy girl, clinging to my arm, and trying to impress me. She even insisted on buying me something to eat. Her flatmate disappeared within half an hour as she apparently felt unwelcome. My girl switched gears afterwards, trying to convince me that she would make a good girlfriend. At least that's how I interpreted it. The person she pretended to be was certainly not the person I met the day before. Among others, for instance, she claimed that she barely drinks and doesn't do drugs. Presumably, she hardly ever has sex either and the box with condoms was placed in her room by her flatmate as a prank.

I want to head home. WILD insists on accompanying me to the station. Okay. On the way there, we walk past a cafe. A woman shouts WILD's name. Who is that? It is TALLBLONDE, giving me a warm smile after saying hello to the two of us. That is unexpected. I really have to get going, though, because it is 3:30 p.m. and I have a date set up for 5 p.m. (Two hours later I already have my dick in her.)

Scrubs

It's the day after. I wake up at around 4 p.m. For a brief moment I question what I'm doing with my life, but this doesn't last very long. I get up and spot a note on my desk that reminds me to contact some girl I chatted up while running some errands in the area. I pull out my phone and text her, "Are you spontaneous?" ER-RANDS replies in the affirmative. We set up a date for 11 p.m. near Mauerpark, which is a large public park in the Prenzlauer Berg district of Berlin. Today is Walpurgis Night, so Mauerpark can be expected to be busy. Funnily enough, I could not get this girl to answer the phone at all. First I called her. She didn't pick up. Then I sent her a message, to which she replied immediately. I thought it's quicker to call, but she once more does not pick up the phone. As this happens, I'm hanging out with my buddy GAMBLE. He tells me about a girl he knows who has the same behavior and who even makes bizarre excuses like writing to him that she can't talk right now because her sister is visiting. We're talking about a girl he was banging and who seemed afraid of using the phone.

A friend from Norway, TEEVSTER, is in town. He's one of the most sexually aggressive guys I have ever met. He's relentless and literally goes from girl to girl. His standards are a bit lower than mine, though. Wait, let's say he has a different taste. Anyway, he gets laid almost every single time he goes out. The difference between him and me is that I go out to enjoy the music, dance, and hang out with friends. Getting laid is a nice and very welcome added bonus. He just wants to get laid. He texts me at 10:30 p.m., telling me that he's ended up at a party full of guys and asks whether I know some good alternatives. I suggest he stick it out for a bit. Well, he texted me again at around 4 a.m., telling me that he has just gotten laid. It's always the same with him.

I head to Mauerpark and show up a few minutes before 11:00 p.m. ERRANDS is nowhere to be seen. I check my phone and see a message from her, which I received at 10:55 p.m. She writes that she is still busy but would join me later. I don't respond and check out the park on my own. On the way, I bump into my flatmate NUMBERS. There are already easily over 1,000 people in the area. I give ERRANDS another shot and call her again at 11:30 p.m. This time she answers her phone. Her voice sounds rather horny. I also get the impression that she is a bit tipsy. With women, those two conditions often go hand in hand.

"I'm still drinking with some friends, but I'll meet you in ten minutes. Stay where you are. I'll make it worth your while later," she pleads.

I have no interest in playing games, so I brush her off and tell her that I'm already on the way to some club. NUMBERS had told me that Bar 25 has its reopening tonight. That's a really sordid place where drug consumption is rampant. Yet, you will find plenty of horny girls there. It's a bit of a problem to find girls who are not too trashy, though. Alas, if you don't want to pay for a cab, it can take quite a while to travel in Berlin. At midnight, ERRANDS calls again, but this time I ignore her. At 12:30 a.m. she tries again.

"Where are you?", she asks.

"I'm on the way to Bar 25."

"Can't you just come back and join me? I'd really like to see you."

She sounds horny as hell — and even tipsier.

"It's a bit too late now. Let's meet up some other time."

ERRANDS isn't worth writing a story about. In short, the next day she texted me, "Are you spontaneous?", at around 11 a.m. I got up at around 5 p.m., so I obviously am not that spontaneous. We set up a date a few days later, hung out for a bit. Then I took her back to my place and banged her.

Anyway, Bar 25 is largely an outdoors venue and therefore only open in the warmer months. It is primarily an after-hours club, meaning that you go there after having been to another club. This roughly works as follows. You party at some club from 2 a.m. to 5 or 6 a.m., but because you are high on coke you can't sleep. Consequently, you party for eight more hours at a place like Bar 25. I'd say I'm one of the very few people going to that place who do not consume drugs.

NUMBERS and I show up at 1:30 a.m. The queue is easily 300 people deep, which does not surprise us. In fact, we are surprised the queue isn't longer. Bar 25 has done a big marketing push for their reopening. Every autumn, they claim they are closing for good, yet every spring they have a surprising reopening party. This year, they had ads plastered all over the subway network. Yes, in Berlin living off welfare benefits and consuming drugs 24/7 clearly has gone mainstream. For that crowd, Bar 25 is the place to be. For their completely unexpected grand reopening they have a really big event set up, running from Thursday midnight to Monday noon. The lineup consists of 50 DJs, none of whom I recognize. In all fairness, though, it is almost irrelevant what kind of music they play as plenty of people only stagger around the venue, looking like zombies.

At around 2 a.m. we have enough of standing in the queue, so NUMBERS and I decide to head to Golden Gate instead, one of the nearby techno clubs. Golden Gate subscribes to the mainstream idea of Berlin chic. Thus, it's a really shabby place. Calling the building that club is located in merely derelict would be quite an understatement. In total, they probably fit around 200 people in there. On the plus side, cover charge is fairly cheap, just around 5 euros. Then again, compared to what you get in return, it may be a bit steep.

We quickly arrive at Golden Gate. Once inside, I bump into a friend of mine, YARMULKE. I want to talk to him, but on the way I spot a rather cute girl. She smiles at me. I smile back. Then I grab her jacket, lift it up and pull it over her head. JACKET laughs loudly and says, "You're funny. Who are you?"

I don't say anything in response but instead cup her left cheek with my hand while making intense eye contact. Then I slowly move my thumb over to her lips. She parts her lips slightly. I put my thumb deep into her mouth, which she eagerly sucks while giving me a lustful look. Both YARMULKE and NUMBERS watch in disbelief. Their expression does not change when they see me successfully going for a make-out moments later. The next day, YARMULKE called me up and said,

"Did I get this right: You walk into a club and within a minute you make out with some girl?"

"Yeah, sometimes it works like that."

But back to what transpired that night. I take my girl by the hand and lead her into the next room. I sit down on an easy chair and pull her down on my lap. We make out again. I pull my cock out and put it in her hands. She whacks me while we are making out. Meanwhile, she has two of my fingers in her pussy. She moans. Then she stops and says,

"Isn't this happening really fast?"

I say nothing. Instead, I pull my fingers out of her pussy again and shove them into her mouth. She properly cleans them with her tongue. She's still working on my cock and is now whacking it a lot faster.

"You really like that, don't you?", she asks rhetorically.

I am getting way too horny and can feel that I'm getting too close to blowing a load, so I put her hand away. Immediately afterwards I ram two fingers into her pussy and hit her G-spot hard. She utters a long, "Uuuuhh ... ." We kiss again. Then I put my cock back into my pants and lift her off my lap. I take her hand and hurry up the stairs to the bathroom stalls. When she puts up some resistance, I stop, push her against the wall and tongue her down hard. I grab the hair on the back of her head, pull her head down and bite her neck. She loves it, but it still isn't enough to get her to check out one of the bathroom stalls together with me.

We kiss some more. Then she asks me for a break. She heads off and disappears to the toilets all by herself. I turn around, wanting to head back to the dance floor. Suddenly someone shouts my name. It's one of my work colleagues. (I started an internship last week.) He's a cool guy but I really don't want stories about my favorite pastime activity spreading at work. He holds a bottle of beer and tells me how "fucking wasted" he was the night before. Funnily enough, Golden Gate is one of the places where people don't really drink but swallow pills and snort a line of coke when they are getting a bit tired. My work colleague seems to think I'm strung out, just like he is. We chit-chat for a bit, then I finally reach the dance floor again.

In order to not squander any more time, I hit on some girl, telling her that I think she's hot.

"What do you want?", she says, in an almost combative tone.

"If you're nice, I'd consider banging you."

She looks at me in disbelief and says, "You didn't just say that, did you?"

"Sure did. How is it going?"

She smiles, puts one hand on my chest and gently pushes me away, but not without saying, "Fuck off, creep!"

That is not what her body language indicated. With one hand I take her wrist, with the other I grab her neck. We lock eye contact. I slowly pull her in. There is no resistance at all. She parts her lips slightly and grabs my neck. She shoves her tongue into my mouth and we are making out heavily. Oh, how her personality changed within moments! Still, I do not like her attitude so I walk off. She shouts, "You better come back later, asshole!", as I turn around to walk into the lounge.

There I run into JACKET again. She stares at me. I walk over and tongue her down right away. She starts asking me questions, but it's too loud in here to properly talk.

"How about we talk outside?", I suggest.

"Yeah, sure."

Minutes later we are outside, looking for a place to have sex. Well, I am. She is just tagging along, asking me where we are going. There are no parks nearby, but I find a nice little unlit area with some trees and scrubs that are tall enough to almost hide us. Now we are standing right in those scrubs. I grab her pussy and rub it. She eagerly unbuckles my belt, pulls my dick out and whacks it. That does not last long because I shortly afterwards turn her around and bend her over. She rests her hands on her knees. I lift her skirt up, pull her tights down and shove two, then three fingers into her dripping wet pussy. I warm her up this way for a while, but not without some objections that went from,

"I have never done this before!", to

"I bet you do this all the time!", to

"We shouldn't do this!", to, finally,

"We can't do this here!"

I'm quite the smooth talker, so instead of addressing her concerns, I say hackneyed phrases like,

"You are so passionate!",

"I love really passionate women!",

"I will make you feel like a woman!",

"You will never forget this!", or

"You turn me on so much!"

I cringe inwardly but keep hitting her G-spot hard. This surely is enough for now, so I pull my fingers out of her pussy and a condom out of my pockets.

"What are you doing?", she inquires.

"You just wait," I say.

The condom is on my cock. My cock is ready and because she has nice long legs, I only have to bend down a little bit to get easy access to her pussy. I put one hand on her flat stomach, with the other I hold the base of my cock. I gently move her back and slide my dick in.

She moans. I put my hands around her waist and want to fuck her properly, yet she freaks out and pushes me away.

"We can't do this here. I really want to fuck you but I am not going to fuck you in public. I'm not that kind of slut."

I stand there with my cock in my hands and nod.

"I have to go inside again. My friends are waiting," she continues.

We fix our clothes and walk towards Golden Gate again.

"Do you mind if I catch up with my friends?", she asks.

"No problem."

Off she walks. I don't know whether this means that I will have to look for another girl. I can't say that I am particularly attached to her, so I really don't care. I watch her walk off. It doesn't take long for some random dude to approach her. His posture is pretty bad and he looks rather meek. He does not look like a threat.

I recall that I have some friends in the venue. I look for them but can't find them anywhere. They aren't outside either. When I walk past a sofa, I feel someone rubbing a foot against my leg. I look down, and it's JACKET who is seductively smiling at me. I sit down next to her. We make out for a bit and then she suggested getting some food together. They are not selling any food in the venue, so we have to go somewhere else. On the way out, I realize that the stamp on my forearm that indicates that I have paid cover charge has almost disappeared. Thus, I take the stamp at the entrance and stamp my arm. The girl behind the till gives me a befuddled look and some guy waiting to pay shouts at me, "Yeah, dude! Way to go!"

We are walking around the area, looking for restaurants that are still open. JACKET clings to my arm and tells me her life story on the way there. I notice a McDonald's restaurant down the street and drop that if everything fails we could always eat there. As I detest fast food, I said this in a mildly cynical tone. Her view on fast food seems to be the complete opposite of mine. She says,

"Oh, a McDonald's? That's great. Let's go there!"

I am not that hungry and don't want to eat anything, so I do not mind. Inside, there is a long queue, which we join. The people in the queue are standing very tightly together, so what better way to capitalize on that than by putting her hand on my crotch? She throws her other arm around me and rubs my junk. Meanwhile, I slide one hand under her dress and play with her labia. This is good fun, but then my phone vibrates. It's BYTE!

BYTE happens to be nearby. I tell him where I am and a few minutes later he arrives at the McDonald's restaurant. As he addresses me, JACKET is still rubbing my

dick through the fabric of my pants. We hang out together. Byte gets some food, too, and then we head
back to Golden Gate. Jacket walks in first. When
it is my turn, the bouncer blocks me from entering by
raising his arm in front of me.

"No, you fucking won't," he commands.

I ignore him and try walking in regardless. He pushes
me back.

"Whoa, dude!", I say, looking him sternly into the eyes.

"Sorry, but we can't tolerate when our patrons touch
the stamp. You won't get in."

Fucking asshole. Yet, I better back down.

I shout, "Jacket, came back here!"

She rushes back to me.

"Is there a problem?"

"The bouncer won't let me in."

"What? Why?"

"He says I touched the stamp."

"Well, you did, didn't you?", she says and laughs.

"Give us a moment," I say to the bouncer.

I take Jacket aside. We hug and make out.

"I really can't leave my friends. But give me your number, okay?"

"Sure."

We make out again. She walks into the club. BYTE and I head to Bar 25.

We reach Bar 25 at around 5 a.m. Expectedly, the queue is now a lot longer, but because people are leaving, it is moving a lot faster than earlier tonight. About half an hour later we are finally inside. The moment I make it past the cash register, some girl shrieks in happy surprise, "Christopher! Christopher! Hi!"

Admittedly, my real name is not Aaron. However, it is not Christopher either.

CHRISSY has a seemingly gay dude with her who is not too happy that his female friend has her eyes on me.

GAYLORD shouts, "That guy is just horny. Ignore him!"

"What?" CHRISSY responds. I decide to let them sort out their issues by themselves.

"I mean, he'll probably try grabbing your pussy within two minutes. Just wait, I bet the first thing he'll do is put his arm around you and grab your boobs."

"No, he won't. Besides, I don't want to get pregnant again!"

(What?)

CHRISSY now addresses me, with her arm around GAYLORD, saying, "He's gay but we nonetheless fuck all the time."

I wasn't sure at all what I should believe. In any case, my expectation that I would run into colossal train wrecks at Bar 25 has been fulfilled once again.

"Christopher, do you want to do some coke with me?", CHRISSY asks.

"Sure," I say. Not because I do coke (I don't) but because I'm strangely attracted to find out how much of a train wreck she really is.

Bar 25 has two dedicated stalls for consuming drugs that are modeled after confessionals, which I find pretty amusing. CHRISSY isn't the only person who wants to make use of those amenities, so we have to queue again. BYTE got sidetracked by the bar and shows up next to me, with a bottle of beer. I introduce him to CHRISSY and GAYLORD. Plenty of people want to do drugs in those confessionals, so the queue is constantly growing. This queue moves quickly, though.

The four of us squeeze into one of those confessionals. CHRISSY pulls a small bag of coke out of her handbag, spreads it out and uses a credit card to cut it. She bends down to snort it. Afterwards she cuts another line, telling me that this one is for me.

"Let BYTE have it!", I say.

He eagerly bends down and snorts it.

Line three is for GAYLORD. He gets right on it. There is still one line left.

"You go now!", CHRISSY encourages me.

I turn to BYTE, "How about you take it?"

He smiles, doesn't think twice, and happily takes one for the team.

We sit down by the water. Bar 25 is located right next to a river. CHRISSY slides up to me.

"So, what kind of drugs do you like if you don't like coke? Or did you think my coke was bad? I know it wasn't the best stuff."

"I don't really do drugs."

"Oh! Do you smoke?"

"No."

"How about hard liquor?"

I laugh, "I don't drink either."

She looks me deep in the eyes. "That's all cool, really, but what do you want to do with me later then?"

I smirk.

In her world, sex without drugs or at the very least alcohol is presumably an impossibility. She is clearly into me, but she is a bit too trashy for my taste to pursue her. I excuse myself, turn to BYTE and head to the dance floor with him. There I notice a slim blonde with tattoos and fake tits. She really knows how to pull off the rocker look, with her tight pants, six-inch heels, and skimpy top. She slowly walks past me, I put my arm around her and pull her in.

"Hello, stranger!", she says, slightly slurring the words.

Her hands are all over my body and I take the opportunity to feel her up as well. A few minutes later some guy joins us,

"No hard feelings, but she's my girlfriend. We should really get going."

I laugh, "No worries, mate!"

He drags his girlfriend off who turns around, wistfully looking at me.

Where is BYTE? I check my phone and see that he just texted me, "If you end up banging her, I'll buy you a trophy!"

Moments later BYTE stands in front of me.

"Oh, here you are! What happened to that girl, man? She's super hot!"

"Her boyfriend showed up. But, yeah, she is. She's porn caliber. If he hadn't dragged her off, she'd still be here."

BYTE and I walk around the venue for a bit, talking to a few girls. Most have their boyfriends with them, often even right next to them. To one I say, "Oh, that's your boyfriend? I didn't notice him." She responds by whispering into my ears, "I really wish he wasn't here. Come by again in a few minutes and I'll slip you my number."

Before I could get back to her, though, I saw a girl I made out with some weeks ago. I could have pulled her back then but I moved on to a girl that was more my type and ended up banging that one instead. She rushes towards me, "I can't believe it's you again, Aaron!" While turning to her girlfriend, she says, "This is the make-out guy!", and demonstratively kisses me on the lips, before sucking on my lower lip. "Oh, and this is my boyfriend, by the way!", she says, pointing to some hapless schmuck. I don't want to know what it feels like to have that kind of girlfriend, or to be that kind of loser. I chit-chat with them for a bit, and then they head off again. A little while later, her girlfriend comes back to talk to me on her own and comes on to me really strongly. She's way too wasted for my taste, so I take her back to her friends, who at first think that I am about to leave with her. One of her friends says, "I'm glad it worked out." This causes some awkwardness for that girl.

After catching up with BYTE, I decide to hit on one last girl. I spot a brunette who is dancing with her blonde girlfriend. I walk up to them. Both seem receptive, but as I turn my focus to the blonde girl she says,

"I know you hit on my friend before!"

"When was that?"

"I don't know, some time ago."

I have no recollection of that. It could have been weeks or months ago.

"You hit on her first, so now I can't do anything with you," she claims.

Consequently, I turn to her brunette friend. She has absolutely amazing tits that are very nicely shaped. This is complemented by her round and firm ass.

"Do you mind if I touch your tits?", I ask.

"You don't even have to ask," she replies, while giving me a sexy smile. "Besides, you already have your hand on my ass."

I slip one hand into her dress and massage her left breast. Her breasts are not particularly big, but they don't look natural either. The breast I am playing with feels pretty hard, which indicates that she has silicone inlays. Her tits are a bit too big to be natural anyway, given how slender she is. That brunette would have been quite a stunner: tall, slim, very toned body, long wavy hair, and those fake bolted-on tits. Unfortunately, her face looks busted. Her nose and lip jobs were butchered. As I'm conflicted about her, I take her hand and walk with her down to the river. Instead of sitting down next to me, she sits down on my lap, wrapping her arms around me.

Our hands are all over each other. She leans in for the kiss a few times. I move back. Likewise, I go in for the kiss, only to end up licking or biting her neck.

"What kind of drugs do you do?", she asks me.

"Drugs? I don't do drugs."

"Okay. Then you probably only want to fuck me."

I don't respond. Instead, I build more sexual tension by touching her face with the tip of my nose. Meanwhile, I'm rubbing her crotch. She goes for the kiss again. Yet, I just can't do it. Her face is too off-putting. Her lips look bizarre. A little later, I force myself to make out with her, but I wish I hadn't. Her lips feel what I imagine fat worms feel like. I can't do this.

"I'm really getting tired," I say.

Moments later I get up and collect BYTE who really should go to bed as well. We head off.

"What happened with that girl?", he asks.

"Her? Her body is amazing, but have you seen her face?"

"No, I just kept staring at her tits. What's the problem with her face."

"You don't want to know."

We both laugh. We share a cab for part of the way home. At around 9 a.m. I'm finally back in my room. It's time to get some sleep and I am happy that I am not sharing my bed with some random girl tonight.

No Need for a Room

I have been in a bit of a funk. On the one hand, I crave the validation that comes from picking up women, but on the other, all of this starts to feel like a lot of effort for just sex. If I want to get laid, I only need to pull out my phone and call one of my fuck buddies over. In order to keep things more exciting for me, I have been pushing the envelope. I was simply curious to see whether I could get a girl who was a complete stranger to engage in any kind of sexual activity with me in public, maybe even in broad daylight.

It's the first of May. I wake up at around 1.30 p.m. and recall that I am supposed to meet up with another girl I hit on two weeks ago while I was running some errands. We have met once already, but that day I had lined up another date right after, so I couldn't quite see how far things would go. Anyway, at 2:30 p.m. we meet up in the Kreuzberg district of Berlin. My recollection was that she was pretty cool to hang out with, but my perception of her has completely changed in the meantime. I can barely motivate myself to keep talking to her. To make things more interesting for me, I suggest we go to Viktoriapark. I head straight to a more deserted part of that park. We lie down in the grass in a remote corner. After some chit-chatting I gently push her down. We end up lying next to each other, cuddling. Time to keep going! I open my pants, pull them down and my dick out.

"Put your hand there!", I command.

"Okay."

She's whacking me while we are cuddling in the grass, but she's really clumsy. Because she can't keep a steady rhythm going, the level of my erection fluctuates between being flaccid, having a chubby, and being almost erect.

"How about you suck my dick?"

"Umm ... ."

After looking at me for a moment or two, while whacking me in such an amateurish manner, she gives me a little speech on her views of relationships, which are more than cringe-worthy.

"To be completely frank, I need to feel really comfortable with a guy before I can use my mouth on him."

"Use your mouth, huh?"

"Umm .... I mean, I could do something like this for you after we have been together for maybe five to six months."

"Right."

"But only to do you a favor, like when you've done something really nice for me. Something like this should only be a reward."

"Oh, really?"

"Yeah."

"When was the last time you've had sex?"

"I don't think you ... ."

"No, just tell me! I won't judge you."

"Maybe nine months ago."

I am judging her for that. I would have judged her for any other answer, too. She isn't that bad looking and she seems to like dick well enough. So, I think the issue is more with her than the guys. My dick has turned completely flaccid in her hands and I do not trust her to be able to make me cum. Thinking of how shitty her blow jobs must be, I take her hand away and put my dick back into my pants. Of course, for complete certainty I could date her for half a year to find out how bad she really is, but I am not that curious. My patience with her has come to an end.

Because I'm such a well-mannered guy, I offer to take her to the nearest underground station before I go my own way again. On the way there, a ridiculously hot girl crosses my path: super-skinny, voluptuous breasts, and a top showing some underboob. We make eye contact. She looks at the girl next to me, which I'm holding hands with. I look at the girl I'm holding hands with and think it does not pay off to have manners. At the very least, I am now absolutely certain that she is not what I want, which is hardly a mind-blowing realization. This brief encounter also taught me that despite drowning in pussy, really hot girls still immediately get my attention.

Later in the evening I went to the big demonstration. In Berlin, the first of May is a welcome excuse for the unemployed and economically disadvantaged to wreak havoc. There are well over 1,000 *Antifa* guys around. That is a partly publicly funded group of far-left radicals that has, as bizarre as it might sound, the support of several mainstream political parties in Germany. I can't say I have many sympathies for the political left. However, if you are able to look past dreadlocks or torn clothes, you can find quite a few hot chicks in their midst.

I meet up with a couple of friends. We join the non-militant wing of the demonstration. Yet, that is only short-lived. At one point, thirty Antifa members run towards us, presumably trying to escape from the police that is chasing after them. Being adept multitaskers, those left-wing domestic terrorists smash shop windows and demolish bus stops on the way. That is too much bullshit for my taste, so I head off after the demonstration is officially over. From what I gathered, the Antifas then moved on to attacking the police in formation. Different strokes for different folks, I guess.

As I'm heading to the nearest underground station, my phone vibrates. It's JACKET, the girl I met yesterday.

"What are you up to, horndog?", she writes.

"I'm on the way home. It's been a long day."

"Don't you want to go to Bar 25 with me? It'll be fun!"

I left Bar 25 barely fourteen hours ago and I'm not willing to expose myself to that crowd that soon again. We arrange to meet up near Ostbahnhof, mainly for convenience. I told her to meet me at 10:45 p.m. My estimation for how long it would take me to get there was way off, though, as I only showed up at around 11:15 p.m. I find her sitting on the stairs, minding her own business. I walk up to her. She's happy to see me and does not seem to mind one bit that I am so terribly late.

I sit down next to her and she's very affectionate right from the start, cuddling up to me and then going for the make out. Within moments we are already making out heavily. I take her hand, get up and try leading her to the tracks. My intention is of course to get her to hop on an *S-Bahn* train and come back to my place. She figures out what's up and asks,

"Where do you want to go?"

"I think we should chill out at my place."

"But I want to go out first!"

She insists that she does not yet want to come back to my place. As there is little point in pressing further, I drop that plan and instead try to remember if there are any parks nearby. It seems she is able to read my mind because she says,

"How about we just sit down somewhere outside?"

I take her hand and leave the train station. The surrounding area isn't particularly appealing. Then again, this is Berlin, so you won't find many areas that are appealing. I'm not aware of any nearby parks, but there's a derelict playground with brushes and a few benches. We head there. I sit down and she immediately climbs into my lap and tongues me down. I pull my cock out, put it in her hand and let her whack me. Meanwhile, I have one hand under her skirt, pull her panties down and shove two fingers up her wet pussy. Technically, we are in a public place, but I'd say the area is semi-secluded.

My plan is to make her horny some more, bend her over and fuck her somewhere in public. Unexpectedly, she tries taking the lead by lying down on the bench but holding on to the wrist of my hand whose fingers are in her. By jerking my wrist, she gestures me to keep finger-banging her. I have absolutely no interest in doing that because if I get her off now, she would be a lot less inclined to take my dick. I put my arm under her shoulders and move her into my lap again. My cock is rock hard. It is also covered by her skirt.

I calmly pull out a condom, tear open the wrapper and roll it over my dick. I pull her pants down some more. She stops me,

"Why do you want a one-night stand?"

"I don't. We can do this again tomorrow morning."

I grab the shaft of my dick, put one hand on her lower back and gently push her pussy towards my cock. My tip is halfway in. She gets up a little bit, takes my dick and pushes it towards my belly with the palm of her hand. Her fingers are wrapped around my cock.

"I'd like to fuck you, but, er, I'm kind of in love with someone and it's not you."

What a pile of crap. I try putting my dick in again.

"No, we have to stop. Fooling around is no big deal, but I can't have sex with you. I'm not a cheater."

I nod.

165

She gets up, pulls her panties up and walks off. That's a rather sudden turn of events, I think. I need a moment or two to fix my appearance and walk after her. A little later I manage to catch up with her.

"Don't be weird," I say.

"I shouldn't have done this. I don't know why I even did this."

"Well, obviously because you're a slut with poor impulse control."

I'm kidding. I did not say that. Instead, I said, "No worries."

We walk next to each other for a few minutes. Then we are back at Ostbahnhof train station. We hug but don't kiss.

"Farewell," she says as she hops on the first S-Bahn train that arrives. The doors of the train close. She's gone. That was anticlimactic.

It's barely past 11:30 p.m. and the night is still young. I've been to too many techno places recently, so I decide to head to Bang Bang Club near Hackescher Markt for some indie rock. An added plus is that it's a fairly cheap place. I really didn't want to stay long as I have only gone to bed at around 9 a.m. the day before.

Obviously, I'm a bit early for Berlin standards. Thus, I am not surprised that the place is fairly dead when I enter. It is slowly filling up. Dancing in a mostly empty club isn't my idea of fun, so I sit down on a sofa, minding my own business. I probably drifted off to sleep a few times, too. The last few days seem to be getting to me. I am indeed feeling quite tired.

It hit me that the DJ played the same song twice in the last 90 minutes or so. "Man, you really are in a quality place," I think and chuckle. Me chuckling somehow makes me feel more awake, so I get up and head to the dance floor. It's still not busy, but there are a few more people around. Two pretty hot girls appear to my right. I dance on my own, and the taller one of them mirrors my movements as soon as she notices me. I take her hand and pull her in. We're making out right away. Suddenly, I am feeling a little bit more awake. I drag her over to the sofa where I had taken a nap about twenty minutes earlier. I feel as if I'm operating on autopilot, just going through the motions as I'm essentially half asleep. Part of me just wants to go to bed. My cock seems to have something else in mind, though.

We sit down. I lift her up and sit her down on my lap. She's gorgeous! We continue making out. She's such a passionate kisser. In between we talk a bit. I learn that she's from *Firenze*, i.e. Florence in Tuscany, Italy. Her accent is a bit thick, but as I'm cupping one of her surprisingly full breasts, given her tall and slender body, I think nothing of it. Based on my experience, Italian girls are pretty amazing. In my top 10 of sexual encounters, they are greatly overrepresented. They easily claim three of the top 5 spots.

We keep making out. She stops and looks me deep in my eyes.

"How old are you, by the way?"

"I'm 29."

She giggles.

"I just turned 18," adding after a pause, "and I really like older men."

We make out again.

"Are you staying at a hotel or a hostel?", I ask.

"Hostel. I'm staying with my class and my teacher."

"Really? Is your entire class here in the club?"

"No," she says and laughs, "but my teacher is here. She's pretty cool. She's only 24 and said that we can party all night."

Then she drops that they are leaving early the next morning. They have to be at the airport at 6 a.m. or so. This means that taking her back to my place isn't an option.

Now she wants to go to the other dance floor at Bang Bang Club. It's the smaller one in the basement. There they play electronic music. It is really dark there. I wonder what that girl has in mind. What she had in mind I found out quickly because as soon as we disappear in the darkness, she grinds her pussy heavily onto my thigh. I put her hand on my stomach, under my T-shirt. She interprets this as an invitation to unbuckle my belt and fondle my cock.

Her hostel is in the western part of Berlin. We could get there by cab, but privacy would be a likely issue as she said that not everybody in her room went out. Going to my place is a no-no because her teacher gave strict instructions that they have to stick together. This does not leave me with many options. I'm assessing the situation. The men's restroom is out of the question because there is a security guard right outside. The women's restroom is next to the entrance and in direct view of the girl at the cash register, the girl at the cloakroom, the guy in charge of the guest list, and the bouncer working the door. Consequently, I take her hand and drag her outside. She stops me.

"I'm not sure I'm allowed to do this."

I grab the back of her head and shove my tongue down her throat. We are making out heavily. I stop kissing her and just lead her off. She shows absolutely no resistance. As we walk past the women's restroom, she says she has to use the toilet. For a moment, I'm tempted to just come with her, but that would have been a bit risky.

She's back within a few minutes, wraps her arms around

me and kisses me once more. We head outside. Bang Bang Club is situated close to a river. I lead her to the river bank, which is elevated. There are stairs leading down to the water. It takes a while to get there because she stops me a few times to passionately kiss me. No, it does not seem as if she is able to contain all her pent-up sexual energy.

We sit down on the stairs. I pull my cock out, which she proceeds to whack eagerly. To up the ante, I shove two fingers into her wet pussy and hit her G-spot. She's really wet! This goes on for a while until she suddenly shrieks,

"Oh my god, I have to be back at the club at quarter past two."

I want to pull my fingers out. She grabs my wrist and indicates that I should keep fingering her. Meanwhile, she is rummaging her handbag, looking for her phone. It's 2:10 a.m., which is just fucking perfect. She puts her phone away. "We only have a few minutes left," she says, before tonguing me down hard, grabbing my neck with one hand and my cock with the other. She squats down beside me, bends forward, takes my dick into her mouth and briefly sucks on the tip. Then she whacks it fast for a bit and sucks on the tip in between.

"Do you think you can cum?", she asks me.

"Just keep going!"

She tries making me blow a load, while I hit her G-spot from a somewhat awkward angle.

Her phone rings. She takes my cock out of her mouth.

"It's a real pity, but I really have to head back!", she says.

"Yeah, I know."

"My teacher is calling. Do you want to walk me back to the club?"

I do. Her teacher and about a dozen of her classmates wait outside, all girls. My girl points out the teacher who is pretty hot herself. She doesn't look too different from the other girls, to be honest. As we approach the group, the teacher addresses me and thanks me for bringing back her student. Then she smiles at me and says, "The night is still young. You'll easily find another girl."

We both pretend we did not hear that. I have an arm around my girl, which she lifts with both her hands to free herself. At first I think she's now demonstrably rejecting me in front of her class, but then the opposite happens. She turns towards me, passionately kisses me and sucks on my neck right afterwards — and all of this happens in front of her teacher as well as her class.

"I have to leave," she says, with audible sadness.

"I know."

We exchange contact information.

"I'll be back in Berlin in September. Let's keep in touch," she adds, sounding very excited by the thought of it.

"What's Your Name Again?"

It's the day after, the 2nd of May. I wake up after a good fourteen hours of sleep. I originally had a date for the afternoon scheduled, with a girl I met some time ago. On our second date, we ended up fooling around in my bed, but she insisted that she couldn't have sex because she was on her period. Tomorrow we were supposed to meet up again. Supposed. After breakfast, at around 2:30 p.m., I check my phone. She texted me, "I'm sorry, but you are neither what I want nor what I need right now." I shrug and consequently scrap my original plan, which was to only go out for a little bit tonight so that I would be fully rested for Sunday.

At around 2:00 a.m. I walk into one of those unlicensed techno places in Berlin-Mitte. I can't help it, but I find that scene incredibly pretentious. The current trend for guys is to go out in sweatpants, which makes me shudder. I hang out in there for an uneventful three hours or so, but just don't get in the mood. It's probably because I'm running on fumes. Okay, time to head home! On the way out, I run into a female friend of mine, a DJ. She tells me about her next few bookings, which include a few places I rather like frequenting.

"Put me down on the guest list for Villa," I say.

She then looks at me seductively, or maybe I'm just imagining things, but I'm hearing the following:

"Oh, you want to cum? If you want to cum, I'll let you cum."

I don't say anything. She laughs, then she grabs my neck, pulls herself up and bites me. Then she giggles and turns to scoot off, but not without turning around and shouting, "See you soon, Aaron!" That was unexpected.

I'm walking around the area, heading down Oranienstrasse. There is music coming out of Tacheles, so I peek inside. It seems there is a party in one of the cafes going on. It's a small place, but the music is great. The guy at the door asks me for eight euros, which seems like a lot for such a small place. I bullshit that I only have two euros left. He says, "Okay." I check my pocket and the smallest denomination I have is a five-euro bill, which I hand over. The guy laughs and calls me a motherfucker as he hands me the change. I wouldn't have minded if he had kept the bill.

The dance floor is small but crowded. I mingle with

the crowd and dance. The music is indeed to my liking. All the girls seem taken, but I don't mind. Now one girl shows up in front of me, trying to get my attention. I don't think she's hot, so I ignore her. After a while she buggers off.

I check my phone. It's 6 a.m. already. Suddenly, I spot a super-hot and incredibly short girl. Her skin seems olive, her hair is dark brown. I'd say she's about 5 feet, 2 inches without high heels. She's skinny, short, has full lips, big eyes, and a really impressive pair of tits. She looks amazing. I take her hand and pull her in. She playfully pushes me away but holds on to my hand. I pull her in again. We lock eye contact. Her hands are on my chest and she's grinding her pussy against my leg. I turn her around so that she can press her ass against my crotch and she really gets into it.

In order to mask that the dance floor is starting to get empty, the fog machine comes on. I can't even tell how many people are in the venue, but I quickly realize that the fog makes us invisible. I turn her around and grab her pussy. Meanwhile, she caresses one of my strong arms with her petite fingers. Now she grabs my neck, jumps up and wraps her legs around me. We kiss. In order to move the interaction forward, I walk over to a few chairs next to a table. Her legs are still wrapped around me. I sit down. She just keeps her legs wrapped around me.

"But I really wanted to keep dancing," she protests, while laughing.

We chit-chat for a bit. She's from Turkey; she drops enough hints to make me conclude that her family must belong to the cultural and economic elite of that country. (I don't think you can find a traditional Turkish girl, trying to hook-up in seedy venues in the early morning hours in Berlin.) Within a few minutes, she shares rather intimate details of her life. I find that a bit off-putting for any girl I'd consider for a more serious relationship, but if your goal is to bang a brunette bombshell, it's probably a good sign.

Let's call her AHU.

"Do you have a girlfriend?", she asks me.

"Do you think I would go out, picking up girls if I had one?"

"I don't know. Plenty of guys do."

I nod.

"Anyway, I had a boyfriend earlier this year. Can you imagine that he asked me after four weeks to marry him? This creeped me out so much that I had to dump him right away."

"You mean the moment he proposed you told him to fuck off?"

"No, not *that* quickly!", she says while laughing hysterically.

"Well, you're super-hot, so I can't blame any guy for wanting to lock you down."

"You're really hot, too!"

We make out.

At that point, we have known each other for ten to fifteen minutes, but the hour is late and she seems very horny.

"We have two options: We either go to your place or to mine," I say.

"So there is no third option?"

"No, I don't think there is."

"We can't go to my place, but maybe we can go to yours in a bit."

We make out again.

"I want to drink some more before we leave," she insists.

Before I can say anything, she's at the bar, ordering some vodka. She comes back with what looks like a fairly large glass. Since I don't drink, I have no eye for those measurements, but it looks like a lot.

"We can share this one," she says.

"I don't drink. You'll have to finish it on your own."

"What, seriously? Okay, nevermind."

She downs it but has to do a second take.

It's not a done deal yet. AHU wants to introduce me to her friends, two guys and one girl. TIGHTDRESS is sitting in the lap of a guy she apparently just hooked up with, HOOKUPDUDE. Then there is ACTOR. This guy is famous, at least in Germany, and most certainly in Berlin. He played the main role in one of the most successful German movies in recent years. AHU tells me that he is her best friend.

It's closing time. AHU collects her bag and jacket. I take her hand and lead her out of the venue. The sun has already risen.

"Wait, wait! We can't just leave my friends behind," she insists.

We walk back in. Considering that she readily left the venue with me, I know that I am on the right track. Then things change for the worse within moments. As I walk back to her friends, with my girl having an arm around my waist, a visibly agitated guy marches towards TIGHTDRESS.

"You're such a fucking whore! How the fuck can you do that!", he shouts at her.

"Get the fuck away from me!", TIGHTDRESS shouts in response, with visible distress.

"On Wednesday you break up with Sebastian and on the weekend you're already out, looking for a new cock to ride, you fucking slut!"

That guy is really aggressive. I am not sure what is going happen. HOOKUPDUDE is not one to stand down, though.

"Chill the fuck out! TIGHTDRESS can do whatever the fuck she wants!", he shouts.

"Yeah, she can, but that doesn't mean it's right!"

You know, I think he has a point. Not that those two guys are interested in discussing the issue like civilized people would. I expect them to start a fight any moment now.

"Hey, HOOKUPDUDE, what the fuck are you waiting for? We're leaving!", I shout at him.

"Coming!"

HOOKUPDUDE walks off, joining us. We are about to leave the venue together. This didn't defuse the situation, however. RANDOMDUDE walks after us,

"You fucking whore, you piece-of-shit human being!", he shouts at TIGHTDRESS.

TIGHTDRESS turns around, "You really need to stop. You're not helping anybody right now."

She is in distress. They are standing around six feet apart. HOOKUPDUDE stands right next to TIGHT-

Dress; Ahu, Actor and I stand next to him. The bouncer joins our group as well. I make sure that we do not corner HookupDude. He has enough space to get away, without having to directly face us. Random-Dude looks at us for what felt like an eternity. Then he turns around and shouts, "Fuck this shit!" He walks off. I see him grab a beer bottle. I tell the bouncer that he should interfere. The bouncer remarks that he was just about to and walks up to RandomDude, who smashes the bottle onto the floor. It bursts into shards and splinters.

I tap TightDress and HookupDude on the shoulder and signal that we should head out. TightDress is visibly shaken.

"I need to go to some other place to forget about all of this," she says.

This is a make-or-break point. Her suggestion is to head to Berghain.

"How about we just relax outside somewhere?", I suggest. After all, the sun is rising already. HookupDude, Actor, and Ahu support my suggestion.

We check whether any of the gates to the nearby rental apartment buildings are unlocked. At already the third gate we get lucky. We trespass and sit down in the backyard. Ahu sits down next to TightDress, trying to soothe her. She's calming down quickly.

I am not sure how I can elegantly get out of this situation, but AHU is taking the lead. As I'm a stranger in that group, I sit back and watch things unfold. TIGHT-DRESS and HOOKUPDUDE are now cuddling. We're just hanging out and talking about random stuff. However, all of us would rather be in bed. After around half an hour ACTOR says goodbye and heads home. AHU sits down in my lap, wraps her arms around me and tongues me down hard. Then she walks over to TIGHTDRESS and tells her that she's leaving, too. She walks off. I follow her and minutes later we are on the train back to my place. On the train, she asks me again whether I have a girlfriend, which I deny.

"That's good. I mean, it's not necessarily *good* good, but at least you are not going to cheat on somebody."

At around 8 a.m. we are back at my place. We are getting it on. She blows me to make me really hard. I reach for a condom, but as I want to put it on she stops me.

"I really don't like condoms. How about we do it without?", she asks.

"Are you sure this is a good idea?"

"I have only been with two guys in my life. I don't have any diseases."

I nod.

"What about you, are you clean?", she asks.

"Yes, I am."

"Okay, then let's do it without."

"Are you on the pill?"

"I'm not, but you don't have to cum inside of me."

I would like to say that I wrapped my dick afterwards, but when this spectacularly good-looking girl had me on my back, straddling me, and gently tugging my hard cock with her petite hands, I found myself unable to object.

She raises her upper body slightly, preparing to let me enter her.

"Oh, what's your name again?", she asks.

"We haven't introduced ourselves yet. I'm Aaron," I say and laugh.

"I'm AHU," she replies and giggles.

Then she slowly sits down on my hard cock and says, "I'm pleased to meet you, Aaron."

One of the Biggest Sluts of Berlin

Over the last two weeks I have been hanging out with AHU who treated me like a king. I particularly like that she wakes me up in the morning, after preparing breakfast for us. The many Western women I have met didn't quite invest that much time and effort. Alas, things had run its course. As I was not willing to make her my girlfriend, she eventually stopped returning my messages. In hindsight, I don't think it was a smart decision to not enter a more serious relationship with her, but back then I just was not at that point yet and was more interested in getting laid with lots of different women. AHU has been really amazing and an utter joy to be with. It took me many years until I found another girl who treated me that well.

I didn't go out last weekend as I was hanging out with AHU. I just spent two days in a row with her, but things ended on a sour note, as I mentioned before. It's Saturday. I thought I better stay in and rest. Those plans went out the window when my flatmate NUMBERS knocked on my door. He tells me about his plans for tonight. Since AHU is no longer part of my life and I currently have no fuck buddy to call either, I think that I may as well go out. Well, it's not as if I haven't tried staying in. Earlier I messaged a girl whose number I had saved in my phone as *landing strip*. She gets back to me while I talk to NUMBERS. She asked rhetorically whether I only reach out to her when I want to get laid. Heck, I thought that that was precisely our deal. I show NUMBERS that message. As we're laughing about it, another one comes in. It reads, "Go fuck myself!" NUMBERS is looking at my phone as this happens. He's a bit befuddled, so he looks at my face, trying to figure out how he should react to it. I look at him sternly for a second or two. Then I grin and finally laugh loudly.

"You had me for a moment," he confesses, and laughs as well.

We agree to head to Berghain together later. We both don't think that that place deserves to be called the "best club in the world," according to some DJ magazine, but it's a decent club for sure. Anyway, time for a nap. Chances are high that it will be a very long night.

At 10:00 a.m. I get up and dress up. A friend from London, TERRY, is in Berlin for the weekend, too. We meet up in Prenzlauer Berg at around midnight and hang out for a bit. Things are a bit off between us. He asks me how I'm doing with the ladies. I hand him my phone and suggest going through my messages. This visibly puts him into a pretty foul mood.

"I've been working so hard the last few months that I just didn't have much time for dating," he says as he returns my phone.

"I see."

"My job's been great. I already got a promotion and a pay rise."

Last year, TERRY got a job at a very prosperous multi-national corporation.

"How are things with you, Aaron? How do you make a living?"

I laugh, "I don't! I'm currently interning to get some experience. Otherwise, my family ensures that I'm not starving."

He mumbles something like "loser" or "leech" between two coughs. I don't think TERRY ever forgave me when I told him I don't appreciate him hitting on girls I'm working on. We had a fallout afterwards.

"Alright, man. It's been a pleasure seeing you. Gotta go!", I say, get up, and disappear. From what I gather, he hasn't managed to date a woman below the age of 30 since I left London. If that were my fate, I'd be pissed, too.

At around 2:30 a.m. I'm finally inside Berghain. Queuing for 45 minutes isn't my idea of fun, but you gotta do what you gotta do. I quickly find NUMBERS in the venue. He is talking to some girl that seems familiar. I walk up to them. The girl looks at me, gives me a big smile and hugs me quite passionately. A few weeks ago I chatted her up in some other techno club, I think it was at Watergate. Back then she asked me whether I wanted to hang out at her place and snort a line of coke off her lower back. I thought she was a tad too trashy for my taste, so I didn't take her up on her offer. I mean, not doing coke but taking her home and banging her. NUMBERS doesn't seem to have any reservations. Then again, he doesn't know what I know.

We hang out together for a while and are a bit disappointed that the place isn't very active.

"Aaron, I just checked the listing. The DJ we're here for starts at 9 a.m.," NUMBERS tells me.

"Oh! I'm not sure I'll last that long."

"That's because you don't do coke, Aaron," the trashy chick interjects.

Anyway, the DJ is a local guy named Sascha Funke. I don't really know many DJs by name, though. I listened to one of his sets online before heading off and thought it was decent enough. Well, the problem with those Berlin techno clubs is that they start really late. You can of course hit on girls at 2 or 3 a.m., but chances that you'll pull will be quite low because there are plenty of places that start to get really busy only at 5 or 6 a.m., if not later. Some people deal with this by taking cocaine, others go to bed early, get up early, and head to a place like Berghain or Bar 25 after breakfast.

Another issue is that there is a significant number of people who specifically pay the relatively high cover charge — it's only high for Berlin standards — to dance to whatever some mildly renowned DJ plays. The more well-known DJs, at least at places like the two I just mentioned, tend to play late. At that time, plenty of girls will be severely whacked out, so have fun running any kind of game on them. It's a pointless exercise to hit on girls who stagger around like zombies. On the other hand, you may find some who just took a bit of MDMA. Those are normally good fun and really eager to take dick.

I leave NUMBERS alone with that coke whore and check out the place on my own. It's getting busier. I spend about three uneventful hours chilling out, listening to the music, dancing for a bit, and talking to the occasional girl. Frankly, I kind of miss AHU and thought it was stupid of me to let her go. Alas, that was then and this is now. Still, it's really not often the case that I miss a girl or develop any kind of emotional attachment.

As I'm getting up from a sofa, I notice a very sexy blonde girl. I get a good vibe, so I walk up to her. She seems really excited that I talk to her.

"Oh my god, I can't believe you just came over to hit on me!", she shrieks.

"You're really hot, so why wouldn't I?"

"I think you're hot, too. But that guy over there is my boyfriend," she says.

"Oh."

"Don't worry. Just say hi to him!"

She clings on to my arm and gently pushes me in his direction. I exchange a few words with him. To me, he looks like a spineless loser. He probably has a good job, though. Anyway, his girlfriend is clearly a lot more attracted to me than she is to him. She turns around, wraps her arms around me and grinds her pussy against my thigh.

Her boyfriend walks over, "No offense, mate, but this is a bit much. You better back off!"

"I'm not doing anything. I think you should talk to your girlfriend, not me."

He turns his head to face her. She looks down and mumbles, "Sorry."

I head off as I don't want to get caught up in any kind of relationship drama. A few minutes later, I spot this girl again, all by herself, at Panoramabar, which is the name of the bar opposite the smaller dance floor, one floor above the main dance floor. I think it got its name from the fact that it's shaped like a rectangle, maybe it's even a square, with four long sides. If you are tending bar there, you certainly get a wide view of the dance floor right in front of it. Anyway, she stands there, sucking on a straw.

"Where's your boyfriend?", I ask.

"I wanted to be on my own for a little bit. I'm really sorry for what just happened."

"No worries."

I have a rough idea where this conversation is heading, but I am really not keen on facing an enraged guy inside a club. For a moment, I ponder whether I should exchange contact details with her, but I sense trouble, so I wish her a fun night and walk off.

Half an hour later I run into two girls who seem really into me. As I quickly figure out, they aren't all that hot. Then again, I just spent two weeks with one of the most spectacularly beautiful girls I ever met. Alright, I'll shut up about AHU now. The point is that I'm probably not hungry enough. Otherwise, I would have shown more interest in at least one of those two girls.

As I'm pondering where my life is going, it hits me that the place has turned into quite a cock farm. Speaking of, I feel the grip of a male hand on my shoulder. My initial reaction is that it's that loser boyfriend from earlier tonight. I quickly turn around, with my right elbow raised, in case I have to deflect a haymaker — it's not that guy but some guy with dreadlocks I bumped into a few months ago. I was unknowingly hitting on his girlfriend. He took it really easy, along the lines of, "You got great taste, man, but I got in there first." All of us laughed, including her. I ended up talking to him for about an hour or so; really fun guy. We exchanged contact details, but I never followed up. I think I've been seeing too many girls to devote much time to expanding my social circle. Well, we hang out for a bit. He tells me that his girlfriend left him and added, "If I had known that she was on the way out, you could of course have banged her."

There was one girl I wish I had approached. She was deep in conversation with a girlfriend and I thought I'd try my luck a little later. But later on I could not find her again.

Instead, I noticed Frenchy who is trying to make her way through the now fairly crowded dance floor next to Panoramabar. A guy who is a bit shorter than her walks behind her, holding her hand. As she walks past me, she puts her other hand on my chest and lets it rest there for a moment. I immediately pull her in. The first thing out of her mouth is asking me whether I'm Italian.

"I'm not."

"I'm French, but it's unfortunate that you're not Italian," she asserts and walks off.

I wait for a brief moment, then I take a big step forward, grab her hand and pull her in again. The dude she's with is dumbfounded. FRENCHY firmly embraces me and stares deep into my eyes. I pretend to go for the kiss. Then I grab the back of her head and gently push it down so that her lips get very close to my neck. She gets the hint and immediately starts sucking on it. It's time to seal this one asap. I drag her off to one of those semi-secluded boxes, for lack of a better term, next to the dance floor. Berghain is housed in a former power plant. The box we are in probably contained some heavy machinery at one point. It is elevated, closed from three sides, and open from one side. There are a few of those boxes in a row.

We sit down. She immediately hops on top of me. We are making out. I have one hand under her dress, rubbing her pussy. She's rubbing my crotch. Then a buff, bald, and half-naked guy who looks a lot like Johnny Sins shows up behind her. I have my cock out already. FRENCHY strokes it in an unusual way. Four fingers are wrapped around the shaft, but her thumb is stretched

191

out, gently pressing against the back of the top of my cock. It feels pretty good.

BALDUR kneels behind FRENCHY, yanks her head back and makes out with her. Was that the guy she was with before? She whispers in my ear, "Two guys at the same time, that's my fantasy." I have no idea what is going on, whether she knows the dude or not, or whether I'm only the willing pawn in a sex fantasy she is playing out. In any case, she seems fine with BALDUR taking part in the action. I decide to play it cool for now.

Then BALDUR wants to make out with me as well. I put my right hand on his chest and push him away, gently but determinedly. He grabs FRENCHY's head again and tongues her down heavily. With the other hand he's fingering her from behind. I know this because I feel his fingers entering her pussy while I'm playing with her labia. Meanwhile, FRENCHY is stroking my cock. BALDUR passes her head to me. I don't want to make out with her after he has just pulled his tongue out of her mouth, so I pull her dress down and suck her stiff nipples instead. This goes on for a while. Eventually, I have to stop her because she is getting quite close to making me blow a load, but I do not want to blow a load yet. She only smiles and grabs my dick again. This time she holds it firmly with four fingers, not whacking it, and quickly rubs the tip of my cock with her thumb. That is an unfamiliar sensation for me. Within around fifteen seconds I shoot a big load. As I do not want to ruin my T-shirt, I yank my dick sideways the moment I start cumming and end up leaving some pretty huge cum stains on her dress. FRENCHY is visibly delighted. She gently caresses my cum-covered cock, then she licks her fingers and says, "I love tasting your sperm." We share some intense eye contact.

FRENCHY leans forward and whispers into my ear,

"Could you please tell that guy to leave us alone?"

I grab him by the neck and say, "Mate, thanks for playing, but now we'd like to have some privacy."

"No problem," he replies. We exchange a firm handshake. I think he's a solid guy.

I'm cuddling with FRENCHY. The guy with dreadlocks from before walks by and gives me a curious look. He probably noticed that my pants were pulled down and that my girl is holding my dick in her hand, even though my T-shirt largely covers it. I want to wave him over, but can't get my hands off FRENCHY's firm ass.

"I'd like to lick your cock for a bit."

"Go ahead!", I say while lifting up my T-shirt.

She gets off of my lap and kneels down next to me. First, she thoroughly cleans my dick with her tongue and then she gently sucks on it for a bit. All of this happens pretty much in public. The box-like structure we are in is open to one side and if it weren't for FRENCHY's impressive mane, it would be fully obvious what is going on. Now a well-meaning observer could conclude that it looks as if she pretends giving me a blow job.

After a while she stops.

"That was good. How about we go somewhere else?", I say.

"I think I should find my friends," she claims.

"Sure. We'll go look for them together."

I take her hand and drag her down the hallway to the bathroom. Moments later we're inside.

"No, this is the men's restroom. I can't do this."

We walk out of the restroom area again. At Berghain, the restrooms are all unisex, but since there is such a surplus of men, you could be forgiven for thinking that the restroom area we were just in is the men's restroom. Berghain is quite a cock farm tonight.

"Girls use that bathroom too, by the way. It's unisex," I explain.

"No way!"

"Just wait, there will be some girls walking in."

About two or three minutes later the first girl walks past us and enters one of the stalls.

FRENCHY looks at me and says, "OK, let's go."

We enter the restroom and luckily find an open stall immediately. I usher her in. She comments on how dirty the stall is. It really is.

"I don't want to sit down on the toilet. It looks gross," she objects.

I nod and pull down her panties nonetheless. One of her arms is around my neck. She keeps it there while bending her upper body down. She starts sucking me off. I have not thought of this position before. It looks pretty trashy. Needless to say, it's also a huge turn-on. She's giving me a good slobbering blow job. I want to do something for her, too, so I enter her pussy from behind with two fingers.

After a good deep-throat she takes my dick out of her mouth and looks at me.

"I don't want to have sex," she exclaims.

"I don't want to have sex either," I respond and gently shove her head towards my cock again.

She's really amazing at sucking dick. I don't want to know how many dicks she has practiced her art on. She continues and takes my dick in all the way. She pulls my pants and boxers down to get better access to my balls. Now I'm getting a deep-throated blow job. Simultaneously, she is playing with my balls. She's really good at the latter, too.

Eventually, she sits down on the toilet seat. I guess it's

no longer gross to her. Probably it was too demanding to suck me off in that rather uncomfortable position she has been in.

"I like what you're doing, but I came about half an hour ago. I don't think I can cum again so soon."

"You just let me do my thing."

She is taking her time, treating my dick very well with her tongue. Not only is she great with her mouth, she also knows how to tease me. She takes my dick out of her mouth, sticks her tongue out and licks my balls. Then she sucks on my balls while whacking me. This she follows up by first licking my balls with the tip of her tongue, then moving her tongue slowly all the way up my shaft. After reaching the tip of my cock with the tip of her tongue, she takes a break and looks at me. I look at her expectingly. She opens her mouth and quickly takes my dick in, all the way. Her lips hit my trimmed pubic hair.

"Your balls are so big. I want to empty them for you," she says after a few thrusts with her head.

She's taking my dick deep into her mouth again. I moan. I can feel that she's getting somewhere. I'm indeed getting ready to cum again. Now she opens her mouth wide. She plunges with her mouth on my cock and makes gargling sounds. She comes up for air.

"I made you blow a huge load before, but there is more

left in your big balls. I'll get it out for you."

She takes my dick all the way in again.

What she is doing is really hot. She now tugs on my balls. I feel her tongue pressing firmly against my shaft as she quickly moves her head back and forth. This is interspersed with her sucking hard on the tip of my cock. It was bound to happen. I blow another load, this time in her mouth. She does not stop. Her lips are wrapped around the tip of my cock, and she keeps sucking as I'm cumming. After a while, I have to gesture her to stop as the tip of my cock is getting too sensitive.

She licks my cock up and down some more. I gesture her to get up. We hug and kiss for a bit. No, I did not use my tongue when kissing her.

"I want to leave now. Can you stay back for a while and let me get out of this stall first?"

"I think it's better if I get out first. Just follow me," I suggest.

Moments later we are out in the hallway.

"I really have to find my friends now," she says.

"Let's sit down for a bit."

I take her hand and lead her over to a sofa. I sit down and pull her into my lap. She wraps her arms around me. We cuddle for a bit. After the people sitting next to us have left, she lies down and rests her head in my lap. Then she puts her jacket on her loins, takes my hand and puts it on her panties. Her jacket and dress will probably accentuate what I'm about to do more than they hide my actions. Either way, I slide my fingers into her panties, but then I tease her a little by pulling my hand out and rubbing her crotch, with her panties separating my hand from her pussy. She moans and arches her back ever so slightly. I take my sweet time doing that. She gets hornier and hornier.

This goes on for around ten minutes. I enjoy watching her arch her back lustfully and moaning lightly. She wants more, though. She takes my hand and forcefully shoves it into her pants. I feel that she is dripping wet. Okay, time to get this started. I could not slide a finger in deep, due to our position, but I still get somewhere. I rub my middle finger against the walls of her vagina, roughly where her G-spot is. Due to the angle of my hand I can't apply proper pressure, which does not seem to bother her too much. What I'm doing is apparently pretty effective. As this gets uncomfortable after a while, I pull my middle finger out of her tight dripping cunt and rub her clit instead.

All of this happens out in the open. The sofa we are sitting on is in a hallway connecting Panoramabar with the unisex toilets as well as another bar. It is also on the way to the smokers' lounge. This means that there are constantly people walking past us. This seems to only turn FRENCHY on even more, judging from how rhythmically she moves her pelvis in response to me massaging her genitals. She takes my other hand and starts sucking on my fingers one by one while moaning in between.

Then she gives me a horny look. She unbuckles my pants, pulls the zipper down and fishes for my cock. Being a true gentleman, I pull it out for her. She licks the tip of it enthusiastically. This is getting a bit too much, as there are dozens of people around us, so I take off my scarf and try covering her head. That doesn't help much. She looks at me while sucking on the tip of my semi-erect dick. She winks at me, then takes it all the way in. Now she slowly and very deliberately moves her head. Her tongue is firmly pressed against my shaft, sliding back and forth. My cock leaves her mouth only minimally, so adept is she at administering those slow and very precise movements with her lips, tongue, and head. Meanwhile, I think that getting blown in public in a busy club is quite something. You need a very special kind of woman for that.

She keeps sucking my dick. I have blown a load twice within the last two hours, so I really am not sure that I can cum again. However, FRENCHY seems to enjoy that challenge. She just keeps going. I can't say that I dislike what she is doing. Eventually, and to my great surprise, my cock gets really hard again. She moves her head back a little bit so that she can grab the shaft of my dick with her thumb and index finger. She gently strokes me that way, while running her tongue over the tip of my cock in her mouth.

I'm very hard. Yet, I don't think I can cum in this position as I only get constant but fairly soft pressure. I could of course grab the hair on the back of her head and make her deep throat me, but that would be a tad too obvious for my liking. Those mini-strokes, mini-thrusts by her head, and frequent licks of her tongue are still great, though. Now I want to cum again. I lean back a bit, take my dick out of her mouth, and whack myself very quickly. Meanwhile, she takes one of my balls into her mouth and gently tugs it with a firm grip of her lips. I'm close to the point of no return. I grab the back of her head and pull her off my balls. I can feel that the pre-cum is already on its way. FRENCHY looks at me with an expression full of lust, opens her mouth, and sticks her tongue out. I put my dick in her mouth. She wraps the tip of my dick with her mouth, sucks on it and uses her tongue for added effect. Within seconds I fully erupt. She swallows all of it.

I have just blown a load in public, so I think, "Whatever, I may just get her off in here, too!" It's no surprise that she is very aroused by the whole thing. I put my dick away and drag her closer to me. She sits down on my lap.

"What do you want to do?", she asks.

I don't answer.

I have one hand on her lower back, the other on her chest. I push her down next to me. She's lying on the sofa, her legs rest on my thighs. Due to me pushing her down rather forcefully, her dress moves and exposes her panties. I fix her appearance but transition quickly to grabbing her pussy. I pull her panties down. My index and middle fingers are on her labia, which I gently pull. I take my hand away and put my index finger on her lips. She takes the wrist of my hand, opens her mouth and engulfs my index finger, sucking on it. I pull my finger out of her mouth again and rub her clit with my now wet finger. She's moaning. I apply more pressure to her clitoris, to which she responds by twisting her body and moaning audibly. The music largely drowns it out, but I notice that some people are giving us a baffled look. Some creeps also linger around, watching what is going down. One dude even has his hands in his pants, presumably stroking himself while watching what I'm doing with FRENCHY. I now add my other hand.

I have a job to do. With one hand I massage her clitoris, with the other I hit her G-spot. I am as discreet as I can be, given the circumstances, which is to say not particularly. I think this has been enough foreplay, so

I increase speed and pressure. She gets off quickly. I am quite startled by how loudly she is moaning. She gestures with her hands that I should come closer. I do so. She wraps one arm around me and pulls me in. We are lying on top of each other.

"That was so good. Thank you!", she whispers in my ear.

We lie down like this for a while, until she complains that I start to feel heavy. We sit up. She cuddles up to me. It seems she really likes post-coital cuddling. After a little while, she is falling asleep in my lap. I can't blame her for that. I pull out my phone to check the time. Oh, it's past 9 a.m. already! The DJ who was the pretense for going out tonight should be playing now. I remain seated, with FRENCHY in my lap. From what I can tell, the music isn't even that great, but who am I to complain?

FRENCHY twists and opens her eyes. Then she slides off my lap, cuddling up to me while placing her head in my lap. Moments later she goes to sleep again. I gently caress her head and upper body and start paying some attention to my surroundings, for once. Some girls in the area are giving me rather intrigued looks. They could have noticed that I have gotten sucked off in public and if it's not that, it's likely that they observed me making my girl cum on the sofa.

Oh, there was some woman I briefly made out with

earlier, which I forgot to mention. Back then I said, "I want to dance first, maybe later," and insisted that I give her some space. She is walking past now and seems green with envy. Well, it's your fault, lady!

BALDUR walks past as well, smiling at me. I wave him over, so he sits down next to me.

"How do you know FRENCHY, buddy?", I ask him.

"Her? I don't really know her. I just met her earlier tonight."

"Oh!"

We chit-chat for a little bit as I'm curious to learn more about him. It turns out he's just a tourist who wants to get laid.

Considering that he has met FRENCHY earlier tonight, his behavior wasn't quite as bold as I initially thought. There is of course the big unknown of what he has done with her earlier. It's not inconceivable that she gobbled down his cock in some dark corner or something along those lines. Still, I think it takes quite some balls to invite oneself to join a man and woman who are going at it. I did not get his whole story, but on the way home FRENCHY told me that she did not really know the "dude from the Netherlands." She even asked whether he was an acquaintance of mine. That was interesting! I thought I am bold and daring, but that guy was something else. Then again, if what I have seen of him that night is representative of his game, he probably has been in a few altercations. Someone less polite than me could just have socked him the moment he joined FRENCHY and me in that box earlier.

BALDUR is a pretty cool dude. By looking at him, with his waxed naked upper body, you would assume he is gay. Here at Berghain it is customary for gay men to walk around half-naked. Of course, he's not gay. He's bisexual. Our brief conversation has run its course. He gets up, then turns around to face me. I feel his grip on my neck. He squats down and tries to kiss me. I turn my head.

"Sorry, dude!", I object.

"No worries," he says and smiles.

He leans forward and kisses me on my forehead.

Off he is. It seems that talking to me has put him in a good mood because seconds later he's approaching a girl. He blocks her path. She stops. They make strong eye contact. He puts his index finger on his lips, which seems to confuse her. Then he puts an arm around her waist and walks off with her. Like a lamb, she follows him. This was fairly interesting to observe. I think he is roughly at the same level as me when it comes to assessing sexual interest and availability in strangers.

Twenty minutes later FRENCHY is still sleeping in my lap. I'm getting tired as well, so I lie back. We are now both cuddling on the sofa, dozing off intermittently. After a while I ask myself what I'm doing because whatever I am doing now in this club is pointless. I say to myself that I should either go home and sleep or look for another girl. (I'm kidding.) As it just so happened, a girl in a tight orange dress is walking past, making intense eye contact and smiling at me seductively. I hold up my hand and she high-fives me. She is looking at me expectantly. I am pretty sure she saw me getting sucked off earlier. My first impulse is to go after her, leaving FRENCHY behind. It might have been a better course of action. Yet, that would have been excessively rude, i.e. leaving her on the sofa all by herself, considering how sleepy she is.

FRENCHY opens her eyes again. The girl in the orange dress notices this and buggers off.

"Where do you live?", she asks me.

"Prenzlauer Berg. How about you?"

"Friedrichshain. My place is a lot closer than yours, but it is such a mess that I can't possibly bring you there."

We cuddle and kiss some more. Then I get up, take her by the hand and lead her to the exit. You may now wonder why I did not ditch her. My reasoning was simply that a woman with such phenomenal blow job skills should keep pleasing me. The original character of our interaction was surely one of a quick, racy encounter of two strangers who will go separate ways afterwards. Yet, all that cuddling probably changed her perception of our interaction. Of course, my alternatives were walking off in the venue or, much worse, getting up while she was asleep.

We make it past the coat check. As we are about to step outside, she stops me.

"Wait, what's your name?"

"I'm Aaron."

"Thanks. Now I feel a lot better. I'm Frenchy."

On the way to the train station, she asks me again where I live and how we would get there. Looking at her, or us, reassures me that there is no possible way I'll bring her back to my place. Not that I mind that much what my flatmates think of me, but I have some standards. A woman with messed up make-up – her smeared red lipstick looked particularly bad – and huge cum stains on a black dress does not quite make the cut. I have to suppress a chuckle as I realize how fucked up she looks.

"I think we should go to your place," I say.

"Okay, if you insist. But I don't have any food at home."

She gets two döner kebabs at Ostbahnhof train station, one for her, one for me. As we board the train, she says,

"Well, I guess you'll come back to my place after all."

We get off at Ostkreuz station. After a short walk, we are at her place. She was not lying. Her place is a fucking mess. There are moving boxes all over the place, piles of books in one corner, a collapsed pile of magazines in another. In the living room there is a nice setup with a big TV, two huge loudspeakers, a subwoofer and about two dozen PlayStation 3 video games, some of which are still wrapped. There is something really fishy going on here.

Overall, I'm really impressed by how big her apartment is. It's not only big, it's also really swanky: newly renovated, hardwood floor, high ceilings. She lives on the top floor of a luxury apartment building. The rooms I peek in have at least 1000 square feet put together. The apartment is probably in excess of 1500 square feet in total. Her place is huge for Berlin standards and even more so for someone living alone.

"How are you able to afford this place, if I may ask?"

She looks down at the floor. After a prolonged pause she stammers,

"I, I had a boyfriend for about four months and hoped he would move in with me after renting this place."

"I see."

This is complete bullshit because if you are not independently wealthy or in the top 5% or so of wage slaves, you are not going to find someone willing to rent out such an apartment to you. She did not make the impression that she's making bank with whatever work she does. Of course, she could do escorting or have some other lucrative gig going on. Let's ignore all of that for a moment. Then the problem still remains that her reasoning is utterly illogical because you don't get someone to move in with you by speculatively renting a place that is well above your means. In any case, all of this is more than just a little bit suspicious.

We sit down in the kitchen and chat for a bit, but she seems a bit tense. Moments later she puts two espressos on the table, which she prepared with the help of a fancy espresso machine. (I don't drink mine.) She mentions that she is working as an elementary school teacher. (There is no fucking way an elementary school teacher can afford such a place on just her salary.) I remember that in elementary school children ask all kinds of random questions and imagine the following dialogue:

TIMMY: Miss Teacher, I hope you had a nice weekend. What did you do?

FRENCHY: Oh, nothing. I just sucked the cock of a random dude in a club, and I did not even know his name. And I swallowed. That he left a huge cum stain on my black dress didn't bother me at all.

TIMMY: Um ... . I did my homework, do you wanna see it?

Accuse me of having moral double standards all you want, but I certainly would not want my children to be taught by such a slut. Not that I have any reservations about those sluts sucking me off.

Our conversation takes a turn towards the weird.

"I don't know why, but I sometimes just get so incredibly horny that I don't know what I'm doing," she says.

I nod.

"I mean, in the moment I can't imagine doing anything else, but afterwards, you know, I kind of wonder."

"How old are you, by the way?"

"I turned 33 earlier this year," she reveals.

I'm slowly piecing things together. From all I can tell, she is childless and the reason why she's horny is simply that her biology is going crazy. Her biological clock is ticking loudly. Thus, she is craving so much for cock. It's either that, or bipolar personality disorder, or both.

"How about we go to bed?", she asks.

"Sure."

We head to the bedroom. I feel a bit awkward. She undresses herself.

"Come, get naked!", she whispers tenderly.

I hesitate, but she just undresses me. Now I'm lying in bed with her. She's cuddling up to me. I have my arm around her shoulder. She rests her head on my chest, which I massage. She looks up.

"Say, do you have a girlfriend?", she asks.

I don't, but I don't want to have such a serious conversation right now, so I keep caressing her. She is falling asleep. It's probably around noon now.

I hear noises from which I wake up. She's pacing in the room. I want to close my eyes and go back to sleep. Yet, she's now standing next to the bed and shaking me.

"I think you should leave now," she says.

I'm half-asleep and don't feel too well.

"I'll continue sleeping in the living room. Please show yourself out as soon as you can."

I mumble, "Sure, no problem."

I dress myself and head to the bathroom to take a dump. There, a pile of magazines catches my eyes: politics, economics, business. "There's no way she's reading any of that," I think. I grab one of them. It has the title *Manager Magazin*. I flick through it while trying to squeeze out a number two. Yet, I'm not awake enough to do any serious reading, so I close the magazine again. Then I look down on the cover. Oh, there is an address sticker! Well, who woulda thunk? The address label has her address but the name of a guy on it.

I look at the next five magazines in the pile. It's all the same. A few come with an address label or some kind of insert with some guy's name. I lift up some more magazines. An envelope with a note scribbled on it drops to the floor. The handwriting does not look particularly feminine. It's the same guy's name!

Okay, time to see myself out. I walk into the living room and tell her that I'm heading off. She opens her eyes.

"I don't think I can ever see you again," she mumbles.

"No worries. Thanks for your time."

I take my things, put on my shoes, and open the door. Because I don't want to cause any undue noise, I gently close the door behind me. While I'm fixating on the door, I notice that the surname of the guy whose name I just noticed is on it, to the left of what is presumably her surname. I shrug. Yet, as I sit on the streetcar back home, I wonder how I would feel if I were successful in my job, making enough money to rent a swanky apartment in a very desirable area — and had a cock-hungry slut of a girlfriend who was overeager to please other men behind my back at Berghain and only felt uncomfortable about her behavior once she brought someone home. I think it's pretty great that there are women who suck my dick in front of an audience, but what does this say about the women who are willing to debase themselves to such an extent, and the men who can't imagine that such things happen or, what is worse, that their girlfriends do them secretly?